THE CARE

of the

OLDER PERSON

www.careoftheolderperson.com

CONTENTS

EDITORS/CONTRIBUTORS

Olivier Beauchet, MD, PhD, Professor of Geriatrics, Dr. Joseph Kaufmann Chair in Geriatric Medicine, Director of centre of excellence on aging and chronic diseases, McGill University

Howard Bergman, MD, FCFP, FRCP(C), Chair, Department of Family Medicine, Professor, Departments of Family Medicine, Medicine, and Oncology, McGill University

Ronald M. Caplan, MD, CM, FACS, FACOG, FRCS(C), Clinical Associate Professor Emeritus Obstetrics and Gynecology, Weill Medical College of Cornell University

Abraham Fuks, MD, CM, FRCP(C), Professor, Department of Medicine, McGill University

Serge Gauthier, CM, CQ, MD, FRCP(C), Director, Alzheimer Disease Research Unit, McGill Center for Studies in Aging,

Professor, Departments of Neurology & Neurosurgery, Psychiatry, Medicine, McGill University

Phil Gold, CC, OQ, MD, PhD, FRSC, DSc (Hon), MACP, FRCP(C), Douglas G. Cameron Professor of Medicine, Professor of Physiology and Oncology, McGill University, Executive Director Clinical Research Center (MGH) McGill University Health Centre

Jose A. Morais, MD, FRCP(C), Associate Professor and Director, Division of Geriatric Medicine, McGill University, Associate Director, Quebec Network for Research on Aging

CONTRIBUTORS

Lysanne Campeau, MDCM, PhD, FRCS(C), Assistant Professor of Surgery, Division of Urology, McGill University

Catherine Ferrier, MD, Assistant Professor, Department of Family Medicine, Faculty of Medicine, McGill University

Sathya Karunananthan, PhD, Postdoctoral Fellow, Ottawa Hospital Research Institute

Cyrille Launay, MD, PhD, department of medicine, division of geriatrics, University Hospital of Lausanne, Switzerland

Artin Mahdanian, MD, MSc, Department of Psychiatry, McGill University

Louise Mallet, B.Sc. Pharm., Pharm.D., BCGP, FESCP, FOPQ, Professor in Clinical Pharmacy, Faculty of

Pharmacy, University of Montreal, Pharmacist in Geriatrics, McGill University Health Center

Silvia Monti De Flores, MD, FRCPC, DFAPA, Department of Psychiatry, McGill University

Randy S. Perskin, Esq., JD, Elder Law Attorney, New York

Samer Shamout, MD, MSc, Fellow, Division of Urology, McGill University

Mark J. Yaffe, MDCM, Professor of Family Medicine, Department of Family Medicine, St Mary's Hospital Centre and McGill University

Haibin Yin, MD, CCFP (COE) Assistant Professor, Director of Undergraduate Medical Education, Division of Geriatric Medicine, McGill University

INTRODUCTION

Jose A. Morais, MD, FRCP(C), Associate Professor and Director, Division of Geriatric Medicine, McGill University, Associate Director, Quebec Network for Research on Aging

It is a well-recognized fact that our society is growing older. This aging of the population is observed in developed as well as in developing countries, albeit at a faster pace in the latter. From the days of the Roman Empire to the early XIX century, average life expectancy at birth remained stable at about 45 years. Since then, there has been a progressive increase in life expectancy with the introduction of improved hygiene and availability of food. The improvement in medical care also contributed to improved survival, especially in older individuals with chronic conditions. Nowadays, a cohort of newborns is expected to live an average of 80 years, with an excess of

3-4 years for baby girls compared with boys. The net effect of this increased longevity combined with the decline of birth rates is practically a doubling of the percentage of older adults, to reach about 25% of the population by 2030 in most developed countries. The prevalence of those above 85 years, the so-called "old-old" will in fact triple to attain 8% of the population. According to the World Health Organization, the aging of the population is an unprecedented phenomenon in human history. Although many anticipate this demographic revolution with apprehension, it is in fact a triumph of humankind over the adversities of the environment. Among many societal challenges posed by the aging of the population is a growing prevalence of multiple chronic diseases and functional impairments of older adults, giving rise to the geriatric syndromes, especially in those above 85 years of age. The shift in the prevalence from acute and communicable diseases to multiple chronic diseases calls for a realignment of the healthcare system that was previously organized to treat acute conditions. The solution resides in an integrated and coordinated system that is more expensive than one dealing with short term interventions, although many inefficiencies in care delivery and inappropriate interventions contribute to heighten the cost.

Why do we age?

Aging is a universal phenomenon defined as a progressive decline in the functional reserves of many body systems and organs once an individual has reached maturity, which in humans occurs between 20 and 30 years of age. These degenerative changes in organs are responsible for the loss of adaptive responses to stress and an increased risk for age-related illness and death. The theory of evolution proposes that the natural forces that shaped life allowed aging to occur because it would be better to perpetuate the species by investing in mechanisms promoting a high reproductive capacity in young individuals rather than in bodily mechanisms that would maintain individuals indefinitely but at greater risk of dying in a hostile environment. There are a number of theories of aging organized in several categories, but those gaining in popularity among scientists fall under the mechanistic theories of aging, grouped as the somatic mutation theory and the free radical theory. Both of these mechanisms are likely to be involved in aging as they implicate basic cellular processes and can explain other derangements at more complex levels of bodily organization such as dysfunction of neuro-endocrine and immune systems. The somatic mutation theory suggests that most somatic cells undergo replication and in this process, acquire damage by spontaneous mutations or by exposure to toxic products. The accumulation of damage will degrade cell function, leading to senescence. The telomere shortening theory can be considered as a special case of the mutation theory. The free radical theory explains that life is a dynamic process requiring metabolized energy that generates free radicals as by-products of normal redox reactions, e.g., reactive oxygen species. Such free radicals are the cause of oxidative damage to cell structures and impair their functions. The mitochondrial theory is considered a subcategory of the free radical theory. Although the body possesses many enzymes and surveillance systems to prevent cellular damage and mutations it is not a foolproof defense mechanism, which is in keeping with the theory of evolution.

What is Geriatrics?

The term "Geriatric" refers to old age that in most advanced societies has been set arbitrarily at 65 years. It is of interest that this age limit was proposed more than a century and a half ago by a German statesman, Baron Otto von Bismarck, based on the observations that at that time, life expectancy of civil servants aged 65 was on average only 2 years. He calculated that it would be more profitable for the state to offer them a retirement pension and to hire new, more productive young people. Since then however, life expectancy at age 65 has steadily increased in most developed countries to reach current levels of about 20 years for women and 15 years for men. Thus, even at age 65, there is opportunity to introduce preventive medicine and to educate people to adopt healthy and active lifestyles. At the same time, the prevalence of chronic diseases increases steadily with age, giving rise to co-morbidities and functional decline. Among older adults, 40-50 % have arthritis, hypertension and hearing deficiencies, 20-30% suffer from cardiovascular diseases, dementia, cancer, diabetes, chronic respiratory conditions, lack of teeth and impaired vision, and another 5-10% have strokes, Parkinson's disease and asthma. Hence, concomitant conditions, known as multimorbidity is highly prevalent as are impairments in activities of daily living. For the age group between 70-85 years of age, 25% have 5 or more diseases, another 25% will experience disabilities in basic activities of daily living, while 50% will be deficient in the instrumental activities of daily living. Geriatrics refers to the practice of medicine caring for older adults afflicted with many diseases and functional impairments. Geriatricians and family physicians with experience in the field know that a care plan needs to address not only a specific condition but also the interaction that results from all of them and their combined impact on the patient's autonomy. Fortunately, there is recent evidence from scientific literature that we are aging better compared with the previous generation with a decline in the incidence of dementia and disability. For many years, there was debate about the different rates at which the decrease in morbidity and mortality would progress. If lower morbidity would outpace mortality, then we would age better and into older years whereas the converse would have the opposite effect. These recent findings are optimistic, in that if further confirmed, persons can expect to live longer with less disability.

Active aging

Aging is a heterogeneous phenomenon that is the result of the interaction between the individual genetic background and environmental factors, not the least of which is the adoption of a healthy lifestyle. Certain families are more prone to develop specific diseases but the appearance of many of them can be delayed or even averted by the adoption of healthy habits. For example onset of type 2 diabetes can be delayed or prevented by regular physical activity and heathy eating habits. There are also several social and psychological determinants of health, including education, income, social status, social participation, perceived control over one's life, positive attitude, to name but a few. With so many factors at play, it is little wonder that each individual ages at his or her own pace. Gerontology has classified aging into three main categories: active aging (previously called heathy aging or successful aging), normal aging and frail aging. The distribution of these different types of aging varies according to different criteria but the majority falls within the active and normal aging categories with 15-25% considered to be frail. According to WHO (2002), active aging is the process of optimizing opportunities for health, participation and security in order to enhance quality of life as people age. The word "active" refers to continuing participation in social, economic, cultural, spiritual and civic affairs, not just the ability to be physically active or to participate in the labor force. Older people who retire from work, those who are ill or live with disabilities can still remain active contributors to their families, peers, communities and society.

Contribution of older adults to society

Contrary to common beliefs, many older adults are in good health, enjoying life and contributing to society. Such contributions extend to practically all domains of social life despite the challenge of ageism. At the familial level, older persons through their experience of life are of great support to their middle-age children, in counselling on many matters and in the upbringing of the grandchildren. In many instances, they provide financial support to them. At the community level, other than assisting a friend or a neighbor, they participate in organizing cultural and social events, thus to enriching their communities. Volunteering is definitely another non negligible contribution of unremunerated work of older people for the wider community. We all have had the experience of receiving information at the entrance of the hospital by an older person who is volunteering, but they also participate actively on boards of museums, art centers or charitable agencies, or in directly providing services to youth organizations and to more dependent older adults. By so doing, those engaged in volunteering also benefit from being socially active, since outreach and engagement enhance their own well-being and happiness. Finally, remaining part of the workforce is another way of contributing as well as of maintaining physical, cognitive and mental capacities. Society will need to continue its efforts to allow older adults to maintain their societal role as all derive benefits. The change in policies to make retirement age non-compulsory is a first step since we all age differently. Furthermore, facilitating different types of work and adjustments of schedules will permit older people to remain active and to contribute to society.

References

1. United population world Ageing 1950-2050, Population division, DESA, United nations, 2002, http://www.un.org/esa/population/publications/worldageing19502050
2. Brian T. Weinert and Poala S. Timiras. Invited Review: Theories of aging. J Appl Physiol 95: 1706–1716, 2003
3. Marti G. Parker, Mats Thorslund. Health Trends in the Elderly Population: Getting Better and Getting Worse. The Gerontologist 2007; 47:150–158.

4. World Report on Aging and Health http://www.who.int/ageing/publications/world-report-2015/en/
5. The Chief Public Health Officer's Report on the State of Public Health in Canada, 2010: Growing Older – Adding Life to Years. http://publichealth.gc.ca/CPHOreport

FRAILTY

Sathya Karunananthan PhD
Postdoctoral Fellow
Ottawa Hospital Research Institute

Howard Bergman MD, FCFP, FRCPC
Chair, Department of Family Medicine
Professor of Family Medicine, Medicine and Oncology, McGill University

M rs. Black is a seventy-one year-old widow with four adult children. Her medical history includes mild osteoarthritis and diabetes, for which she takes acetaminophen as required. She lives alone, tends to be socially isolated, and has mild depressive symptoms. She walks without aids but seems to have slowed down lately. Her cognition is normal, and she is completely independent for all instrumental (IADLs) and basic activities of daily living (ADLs).

Is she frail? What is frailty, and can it be identified in the clinical setting? Are there interventions that effectively delay the onset of frailty or prevent adverse outcomes?

Most geriatricians affirm that they can identify frailty in patients when they see it[1,2]. Experts generally agree that frailty in older persons refers to a state of vulnerability to adverse health outcomes. It is considered different from aging per se, since some individuals live to an old age without becoming frail. Furthermore, individuals of the same age can be quite different in terms of how frail they are. Frailty would be the opposite of what many consider successful aging[3].

However, after three decades of research, there remains considerable uncertainty around the concept of frailty and its clinical usefulness. Conflicting ideas abound on the definition of frailty, what criteria should be used for its recognition, and its relationships with aging, disability, and chronic disease[3-6] .

Definitions and conceptualizations of frailty

Most experts agree that frailty is the manifestation of impairments in multiple organ systems that results in increased susceptibility to poor health outcomes[2]. The specific characteristics of frailty, however, remain an important point of contention.

Some have proposed that frailty fits the model of a medical syndrome, whereby all of its symptoms are linked through a single underlying biological mechanism. The most widely used definition of frailty fitting that approach includes five criteria:

1. shrinking (i.e., weight loss)
2. weakness (i.e., loss of muscle strength)
3. exhaustion
4. slowness (i.e., decreased walking speed)
5. low levels of physical activity.

An individual with any three or more of these five criteria is classified as frail[2].

Another widely applied approach is to define frailty as an indicator of global health status, whereby an individual's level of frailty is ascertained through a wide range of factors that may contribute to their well-being. A definition fitting this approach may pull together up to a hundred different characteristics ranging from visual impairment to poor social conditions, chronic diseases, and disability, into a single index of frailty[7]. For each characteristic, an individual is rated as either having a deficit or not. The frailty index is calculated as a proportion representing the number of deficits over the total number of characteristics assessed. By this approach, the more individuals have wrong with them, the more likely they are to be frail.

These approaches represent very different notions of what it is to be frail. The choice of approach has important implications for clinical applicability as well as the potential interventions and prevention of frailty. The number of frailty scores related to these and other approaches is constantly growing. A recent study identified 67 frailty scores with important heterogeneity across scores in the identification of individuals as frail[5].

What can be done about frailty?

Interventions to prevent or reduce frailty have included physical activity, nutrition, memory training, and individually tailored geriatric care models[8, 9]. Effectiveness of these interventions has been mixed and the body of evidence is limited, given that the definition of frailty is not consistent across studies. Furthermore, these interventions largely overlap with those recommended for prevention or management of chronic diseases related to aging. Researchers have yet to establish whether targeting these interventions to frail individuals has added value.

Thus far, research has provided substantial evidence that frailty, however it may be defined, is a risk factor for various poor health outcomes. Individuals identified as frail are more likely to experience medical complications, disability, institutionalization or even death, compared to their non-frail counterparts, especially when exposed to stressors such as surgery, chemotherapy or falls. Based on this, many experts are advocating screening for frailty in all older patients. It has been shown, however, that risk factors that demonstrate high statistical significance may not be good predictors at the patient-level. In fact, very little is known about the contribution of frailty in improving patient-level prediction[10]. This needs to be investigated much further in order to justify the adoption of frailty as a clinical tool.

What frailty means to older persons

Older persons themselves may have their own perspectives of what it means to be frail. For example, factors such as mood, have been cited as important to patients and their families; often these are overlooked by clinicians and researchers[3, 11]. Psychological health plays an important role in older persons' beliefs about aging successfully. In a study of older persons where only 15% experienced absence of physical illness, 92% reported feeling like they were aging successfully[12].

The research evidence has demonstrated that stereotypes of aging, both positive and negative, are internalized by older persons. This can have both short- and long-term effects on their health[13]. For example, when older adults are exposed to negative aging stereotypes, performance on memory tasks, handwriting and walking speed, as well as physiological measures such as blood pressure, pulse rate, and skin conductance become worse. In fact, in one study, the research showed that an increase in walking speed for those exposed to positive aging stereotypes was comparable to that seen with several weeks of rigorous exercise. Negative stereotypes act as cardiovascular stressors while positive stereotypes reduce evidence of cardiovascular stress. Positive perceptions about aging have impressive long-term effects as well. Individuals with positive self-perceptions of aging have been found to have better functional abilities over a period of eighteen years. These findings should serve as a caution about a potential self-fulfilling prophecy when labelling older persons as "frail".

Conclusion

Frailty is believed to be an early sign of declining health. As such, it may serve as a "red flag" prior to the occurrence of more severe or irreversible conditions, such as disability. In the example of Mrs. Black, the family and doctors would want to identify any factors that are contributing to her declining health and then attempt to address these. The goal is to prevent or at least slow down her decline.

However, after decades of research and discussion among experts, we are still far from a unified definition or diagnostic criteria for frailty. At this time, there is still very limited evidence on the added clinical value of frailty, and currently no evidence-based guidance on how to manage, treat of reverse frailty[9].

For Mrs. Black, better management of her chronic diseases and interventions to improve her social isolation can contribute to slowing down her decline. A diagnosis of frailty, however it is defined, is not likely to have an impact on the clinical care she receives and may only cause harm related to labeling.

References

1. Kaethler Y et al. Defining the concept of frailty: a survey of multi-disciplinary health professionals. Geriatric Today: J Can Geriatr Soc. 6: 26-31 (2003).
2. Fried, L. P. et al. Frailty in older adults: evidence for a phenotype. J. Gerontol. A. Biol. Sci. Med. Sci. 56, M146–156 (2001).
3. Bergman, H. et al. Frailty: an emerging research and clinical paradigm--issues and controversies. J. Gerontol. A. Biol. Sci. Med. Sci. 62, 731–737 (2007).
4. Hogan DB, MacKnight C, Bergman H. Models, definitions, and criteria of frailty. Aging Clin Exp Res. 15(Suppl 3):1–29 (2003).
5. Aguayo GA et al. Agreement Between 35 Published Frailty Scores in the General Population. Am J Epidemiol. 186(4):420-434 (2017).
6. Sternberg SA, Wershof Schwartz A, Karunananthan S, Bergman H & Clarfield AM. The identification of frailty: a systematic literature review. J. Am. Geriatr. Soc. 59: 2129–2138 (2011).

7. Rockwood, K. & Mitnitski A. Frailty in relation to the accumulation of deficits. J. Gerontol. A Biol. Sci. Med. Sci. 62: 722-7 (2007).

8. Puts MT et al. Interventions to prevent or reduce the level of frailty in community-dwelling older adults: a scoping review of the literature and international policies. *Age and Ageing.* 46(3): 383–392.

9. Walston J, Buta B, Xue QL. Frailty Screening and Interventions: Considerations for Clinical Practice. Clin Geriatr Med. 34(1):25-38 (2018).

10. Sourial, N. et al. Implementing frailty into clinical practice: a cautionary tale. J. Gerontol. A Biol. Sci. Med. Sci. 68: 1505-11 (2013).

11. Grenier, A. & Hanley, J. Older Women and 'Frailty' Aged, Gendered and Embodied Resistance. Curr. Sociol. 55: 211–228 (2007).

12. Montross, L. P. et al. Correlates of self-rated successful aging among community-dwelling older adults. Am. J. Geriatr. Psychiatry Off. J. Am. Assoc. Geriatr. Psychiatry 14: 43–51 (2006).

13. Richardson, S., Karunananthan, S. & Bergman, H. I May Be Frail But I Ain't No Failure. Can. Geriatr. J. CGJ 14: 24–28 (2011).

DOCTOR, MY WIFE IS GETTING FORGETFUL

Serge Gauthier, C.M., C.Q., MD, FRCPC
Director, AD Research Unit, MCSA
Professor, Departments of Neurology & Neurosurgery, Psychiatry,
Medicine, McGill University
McGill Center for Studies in Aging

Exemplary case

A 78 year old lady is accompanied by her husband and daughter. The family is concerned about a memory decline over the past two years, worse the past six months. For example she forgets conversations, is losing interest in going out, and was twice late paying some household bills. She does not appear concerned about any of this. The family wants to know if this is early dementia and what can be done about it.

On further questioning she has forgotten some of the grandchildren's birthdays in the past year, is looking for things in the house and gets upset about it. She cooks only simple meals and gets flustered when her daughter's family is visiting. She drives in familiar areas, mostly to visit her daughter. The husband has taken over most of the household finances through their common bank account. There is no advanced power of attorney for medical and financial decisions. She is independent for self-care. Her medical history is of mild labile arterial hypertension, controlled by a diuretic. She takes vitamin D supplements on a weekly basis. Her mother died of Alzheimer's at age 85.

The physical examination showed a pleasant and healthy looking elderly woman. Her Mini Mental State Examination (MMSE) is 21/30, with wrong day, date, month, year, name of the clinic, forgetting 3 words after distraction, unable to copy the drawing. She is unable to complete the short version of Trail B found in the Montreal Cognitive Assessment (MoCA), and to set the time at 11:10 on her clock.

The initial clinical impression is of a dementia due to Alzheimer's disease (AD). A head un-infused ("plain") head computer tomography showed generalized atrophy compatible with the age of the patient.

At the follow-up visit the MMSE score was 20, and the diagnosis of AD was disclosed to the patient and the family. A road test by an occupational therapist and an advance power of attorney to be drawn by a legal professional were recommended. A cholinesterase inhibitor (CI) was prescribed.

General work-up and diagnostic recommendations

Screening for cognitive decline in older persons without symptoms using tools such as the MMSE and the MoCA is not recommended in routine clinical practice. When symptoms suggestive of a progressive cognitive decline are spontaneously brought forward by reliable family members, there has to be a systematic assessment. First a semi-structured questionnaire about the types of cognitive symptoms (memory, language, orientation, judgment), how they affect daily life, and if they are accompanied by mood, personality or behavioral changes, is utilized. Then a general physical examination and a basic neurologic examination are done, looking for evidence of factors that may suggest a vascular etiology to the cognitive decline. For instance systolic hypertension associated by an asymmetry of deep tendon reflexes and of plantar responses would suggest a silent stroke.

The latest (4th) Canadian Consensus Conference on the Diagnosis and Treatment of Dementia published in 2012 an update of its recommendations reiterating that structural imaging using computer tomography (CT) or magnetic resonance imaging (MRI) is needed in a specific set of circumstances (Table 1).

TABLE 1: Recommendations from the CCCDTD about structural imaging needed if cognitive decline and:
• age less than 65
• rapid (1 or 2 months) unexplained decline in cognition and function
• short duration of symptoms (less than two years)
• recent and significant head trauma
• unexplained neurological symptoms such as headaches or seizures
• history of cancer
• use of anticoagulation or history of bleeding disorder
• early urinary incontinence and gait disorder
• lateralizing signs (hemiparesis, unilateral grasp or Babinski)
• prominent gait disturbance

The most common finding on CT or MRI in persons with mild dementia is generalized atrophy, which may be asymmetric, and is compatible with AD. Small (lacunar) infarcts may be found, and are not considered clinically significant towards the cognitive decline unless they are in a strategic area of the brain such as the thalamus or the head of the caudate, in which case a mixed etiology (AD and stroke) dementia is diagnosed.

The other relatively common type of late-onset dementia is Lewy Body (DLB), a mixture of AD and Parkinsonian features, which translates into visual hallucinations early in the course of the cognitive decline, fluctuations of symptoms from hour to hour, and motor changes such as rigidity with cogwheeling (the racket-like feeling when manipulating the neck or arms of a patient).

General treatment considerations

An accurate diagnosis of dementia can be made by all clinicians if there is reliable historical information, some basic cognitive tests and structural brain imaging when appropriate. The etiology of the dementia over age 75 is essentially, AD, AD with stroke, AD with some Parkinson features, or DLB.

What is not as easy is the disclosure of the diagnosis which should be as transparent as for someone with cancer. Most patients with dementia have relative indifference (anosognosia) to their symptoms and to their cause, but clinicians should be on the look out for someone with depressive symptoms. Practically speaking, the accompanying family member should be made aware of the diagnosis and potential consequences on driving and managing finances. If the patient asks he can be told about being in "early stages of a common brain aging condition", and if he specifically asks about AD tell the truth about the likelihood of this specific diagnosis (80% accuracy using clinical diagnosis) unless there is concern for a catastrophic reaction, which is very uncommon.

The loss of autonomy for instrumental and basic activities of daily living is progressive over many years, best handled by gradual adjustments of the family, and is facilitated by support groups. There is no need to make a list of all the changes to occur over five years at the time of diagnosis, but is it wise to anticipate losses though the annual or bi-annual follow-ups: driving, banking, cooking, traveling on foot, day programs, long term care, end-of-life care will be handled over time.

The mood and behavioral symptoms of dementia are often worse that the cognitive decline and the gradual loss of autonomy. Apathy, irritability and suspiciousness are common in the early stages of AD, and may be helped by antidepressants acting on serotoninergic pathways. Hallucinations in DLB improve with CIs. Aggressive behavior not manageable by environmental non-pharmacological approaches may require an atypical neuroleptic such as risperidone (attention to the black box warning about increased risk of stroke and death). Sometimes aggressive behavior is improved by antidepressants and/or the NMDA receptor antagonist memantine, reducing the need or the dose of a neuroleptic.

References

1.   Gauthier S, Patterson C, Chertkow H et al. 4th Canadian Consensus Conference on the Diagnosis and Treatment of Dementia. Can J Neurol Sci 2012; 39: Suppl 5:

HOW TO DIAGNOSE AND MANAGE DELIRIUM

By Haibin Yin, MD, CCFP(COE),
Assistant Professor, Director of Undergraduate Medical Education,
Division of Geriatric Medicine, McGill University

Clinical vignette

An 84-year-old female living at home with mild mixed dementia and Parkinson's disease was admitted for right intertrochanteric fracture after a fall. Functionally, she required assistance for most instrumental activities of daily living, and could perform most basic activities of daily living. She had 24-hour private help at home.

Her past medical history included congestive heart failure, Parkinson's disease and atrial fibrillation on Coumadin. On POD #2, she began to have visual hallucinations and became disoriented. She also had delusion of persecution.

Her mental status fluctuated, from trying to get out of bed to sleepiness. She refused to eat and to take her medications.

She was in abdominal restraints. She was alert and calm, but hesitated for 15 seconds or more to answer questions. Her vital signs were normal. There were no additional heart sounds. Her JVP was slightly elevated. Her lung examination revealed decreased air entry bilaterally. Her abdomen was soft and bowel sounds were present. Her wound was clean with no surrounding edema. Both lower extremities were edematous (R>L) but non-tender. There were no neurovascular damages distally. She had bilateral upper extremity resting tremors and cogwheeling rigidity.

Her medications included Morphine 1.25mg SQ q 2 hours PRN (non-taken in past 24 hours), Haldol 0.5mg IM tid PRN (received 2 doses in past 24 hours), Sinemet 100/25 1 PO tid, Coumadin 5mg PO qd with Lovenox (prophylactic dose) bridging and Lasix 20mg PO bid. What could be the potential causes of this patient's delirium and how should it be managed?

What is delirium? Why is it important to recognize it?

Delirium is also known as acute brain failure, toxic-metabolic encephalopathy or acute confusional state. DSM-V defines it as acute changes (with fluctuating course) in attention, awareness and cognition, that are caused by an underlying medical condition or medication. Different studies show that it affects one third of patients over 70 years old on general medical units, amongst which half are delirious on admission. Among geriatric patients in the Emergency Room, 15% are delirious. In the ICU, prevalence could reach 70%.

The most useful tool for diagnosing delirium is the Confusion Assessment method (Table 1). This systematic-review-validated tool reaches sensitivity and specificity of over 90%. It has also been adapted for patients in the ICU (CAM-ICU). Other tools (Delirium Symptom Index, The 4-AT Test etc.) could also be used.

The pathophysiology of delirium is poorly understood. Several hypotheses include primary or secondary neuroinflammation and cholinergic deficiency. The predisposing factors of delirium include old age, functional impairment, cognitive deficits, multiple medical comorbidities and sensory impairment. The precipitating factors can include many medical conditions, medications and interventions (restraints, indwelling devices etc.).

TABLE 1: Confusion Assessment Method (Positive if criteria 1,2,3 or 1,2,4 are present)
1. Acute change in mental status from baseline and fluctuation in behaviour during the day, AND
2. Attention impaired, easily distractible, difficulty keeping track of what is being said, AND
3. Disorganized/incoherent thinking or illogical conversation, OR
4. Altered mental status (hyperalert, lethargic, difficult to arouse)

One of the reasons why it is important to recognize and manage delirium is its poor outcome. A meta-analysis which follows 3000 patients for 2 years showed that delirium was associated with a 2-fold increase in death, 2.4-fold in institutionalization and 12.5-fold in new dementia. Despite traditional view that delirium was a transient and reversible condition, recent evidence has shown that persistence of delirium occurs in many patients, and is associated with poor long-term outcomes.

Unfortunately, despite this, delirium is often under-recognized by physicians. Several factors could explain this reality. Firstly, hyperactive delirium, which is the most noticeable subtype, represents only 25% of the cases. Hypoactively delirious patients attract less attention of the medical team, despite their poorer prognosis. Secondly, physicians often have a snapshot of their patient once per day, however, by definition, delirium is a fluctuating syndrome. Thirdly, diagnosing delirium could be time-consuming as it often involves detailed interview with collateral historians as well as chart reviews to identify the acute change and fluctuation. Finally, in some cases, delirium could be difficult to distinguish from other conditions, such as Lewy Body dementia, depression and mania. Therefore, clinicians should always have a high index of suspicion and be diligent in their assessments.

What are the causes (precipitating factors) of delirium? How to investigate?

The causes of delirium are vast. Any acute medical illness or medication can precipitate delirium. Infections are the most-commonly diagnosed. Any infection has the potential of being the underlying cause. The presence of asymptomatic bacteruria, however, often leads to a misdiagnosis of UTI causing delirium. Recent studies show that antibiotic therapy in these patients does not change the course of delirium. Electrolyte imbalances, especially of sodium, calcium and glucose, could cause delirium. Cortisol excess or insufficiency could be manifested as hyperactive and hypoactive delirium, respectively. In patients with history of falls presenting with delirium, intracranial bleeding should be considered in the differential diagnosis. In patients with hypoactive delirium, particular attention should be paid to rule out hypoxia and CNS infections. In patients with cirrhosis, hepatic encephalopathy should be ruled out. Hypoxia or shock due to any cause could cause acute confusion due to brain hypoperfusion. In patients that develop delirium days after admission, alcohol or benzodiazepine withdrawal should be considered. Other precipitants include physical restraints, indwelling devices (Foley catheters, central venous catheters etc.), immobility, urinary retention, fecal impaction and uncontrolled pain.

Many medications can precipitate delirium. Common candidates are benzodiazepines, opioids, anticholinergics, antiparkinsonians, antipsychotics, antidepressants (especially TCAs and MAOIs) and NSAIDs.

In order to summarize the above precipitants, the following mnemonics provided by Wise, M.G. (1986) is helpful (Table 2):

Taking history of delirium (mostly taken with the collateral historian) should include a detailed timeline of the acute confusion as well as symptoms leading to or co-occuring with the onset of the acute confusion. A detailed review of systems could help diagnose the underlying causes of delirium. A thorough medication review is important not only for deciphering changes that can contribute to the acute confusion, but also for addressing polypharmacy which could potentially prolong and exacerbate delirium. Past medical history can also provide cues because acute exacerbation or decompensation of many chronic medical conditions could lead to delirium.

On physical examination, the general appearance can provide information such as hydration status, nutritional status, attention and sensorium. Special attention should be given to vital signs. For example, hypotension and tachycardia could indicate ischemia, sepsis or severe dehydration. Fever could indicate infection or pulmonary embolism. Desaturation could indicate cardiac and pulmonary causes. A thorough physical examination should be focused on the potential underlying acute medical conditions. A well-documented mental status examination could help clinicians track the evolution of delirium. If possible, a mini-mental status examination could be done to quantify the cognitive changes during delirium, which could serve the purpose of a point of comparison when delirium improves in the future.

TABLE 2: Causes of delirium – I WATCH DEATH	
I	–	infectious: pneumonia, UTI, CNS infections, abscesses, osteomyelitis, endocarditis etc.
W	–	withdrawal: from benzodiazepines, alcohol
A	–	Acute metabolic changes: acidosis/alkalosis, hypo/hyperNa, hypo/hypoCa, acute kidney and liver failure
T	–	Trauma: Intracranial bleeding, brain injury
C	–	CNS pathology : Intracranial tumor, post-ictal state
H	–	Hypoxia : Anemia, pulmonary embolism, CHF, myocardial infarctions
D	–	Deficiencies: Vitamin B1, B12
E	–	Endocrine: hypo/hypercortisol, hypoglycemia
A	–	Acute vascular : hypertensive emergency, stroke
T	–	Toxins and drugs : benzodiazepines, opioids, anticholinergics
H	–	Heavy metals

What initial investigations should be requested for delirium?

Investigations should include basic laboratory tests, including complete blood count, biochemistry profile (including urea, creatinine, calcium and magnesium), glucose, coagulation profile, TSH, Vitamin B12, and liver function tests. An EKG could be ordered, not only to identify potential cardiac causes if indicated by history, but also to document baseline QTc, as many medications (including antipsychotics and antibiotics) have potential to cause QTc prolongation.

Other investigations may be required depending on the history and examination. If the patient is febrile, septic work-up (blood cultures, urine analysis and culture, CxR etc.) should be ordered before starting antibiotics. If there is suspicion of meningitis or encephalitis, a lumber puncture should be done. Urine or serum toxicology should be ordered if there is suspicion of medication, alcohol and drug toxicity. For patients with suspicion of hypoxemia, hypercapnia or shock, arterial blood gas and lactate could be ordered. If cardiac ischemia is suspected, serial troponins should be ordered. For patients with history of falls, CT-head should be considered. For patients with suspicion of urinary reten-tion, a post-void residual should be obtained.

Table 3 summarizes initial work-up for patients with delirium.

TABLE 3: Investigations for delirium	
Essential	CBC, SMA-10, glucose; INR, PTT; TSH; Vitamin B12, LFTs, ECG
May be required	Blood cultures x 2, Urinalysis and culture, Urine toxicology Lactate, Venous Blood Gas, Serial Troponins, EtOH level
	Post-void residual, Tot & conj Bilirubin, Albumin, Amylase CT-head, Chest X-ray

How to manage delirium

Most patients with delirium require hospitalization, not only for investigation and medical therapy purposes, but also for behavioral management, to manage acute functional deficits, to manage complications and for rehabilitation. For the management of neuropsychiatric symptoms of delirium, a non-pharmacological approach is favoured. For aggressive patients, distraction and de-escalation strategies should be adopted. For patients with day-night reversal, it is important to promote good sleep hygiene by ensuring adequate light during the day and darkness at night. For all patients with delirium, physical restraints should be avoided, as they not only prolong delirium and cause immobilization syndrome, but also increase risk of strangulation. Ensuring proper hydration and nutrition could prevent delirium from worsening. It is also important to monitor and prevent the development of pressure ulcers. It is important to compensate for patients' sensorial deficits, by encouraging uses of glasses and hearing aids. Orientation cues such as photos of family members and calendar, should be used if possible. Early mobilization could be helpful to prevent deconditioning and immobilization syndrome. Occupational therapy assessments are helpful for discharge planning purposes when delirium improves.

When and how to use medications for behavioral disturbances?

Non-pharmacological approaches should almost always be attempted first to curb agitation. One of the only circumstances where pharmacological approaches should be used first is if the patient's agitation poses a risk of self-harm or a threat to others.

Antipsychotics such as Haloperidol, Quetiapine, Risperidone, Olanzapine and Ziprasidone are first-line pharmacological treatments for agitation in delirium. Haloperidol is the most efficient against aggression, however, high doses of haloperidol (>4.5mg per day) are associated with an increase in extrapyramidal side effects. Based on limited evidence, it is recommended that low-dose haloperidol (0.5mg to 1.0mg PO or IM) should be used for the control of agitation and psychotic symptoms, up to a maximum of 3mg per day. Its onset is 30 to 60 minutes after parenteral administration, longer if PO. Please note that IV haloperidol should be avoided due to QTc prolongation. Seroquel is the most sedating antipsychotic, and causes less extrapyramidal signs and symptoms. Its main limitation is that it can only be given per os. Its starting dose is 12.5mg to 25mg with a maximum dose of 50mg per day.

It is worth mentioning that a recent meta-analysis of randomized trials showed that antipsychotics do not alter the duration or severity of delirium, and do not reduce ICU admissions or mortality. Therefore, clinicians should be cautious when prescribing antipsychotics, by weighing apparent benefits with the risks of antipsychotic side-effects and complications (i.e. falls, stroke, increased mortality).

Benzodiazepines are second-line agents, due to respiratory depression, paradoxical excitation, fall risk and oversedation. However, benzodiazepines such as Ativan could be used first-line in specific situations where antipsychotic use should be avoided. These include patients with seizures, in those in alcohol or benzodiazepine withdrawal, and in those with a history of neuroleptic malignant syndrome or Lewy Body Dementia (who are very sensitive to antipsychotics).

Benadryl, Gravol and other medications with significant anticholinergic effects should be avoided, as they may exacerbate and prolong delirium.

All medications for agitation should be discontinued as soon as possible and should usually not be continued beyond the hospitalization for delirium. In the minority of patients who require antipsychotics on discharge, caution needs to be exerted so that the prescription has a finite duration and should be reassessed frequently with appropriate follow-up.

Table 4 summarizes the above choices of initial pharmacological regimen.

TABLE 4: Pharmacological management of hyperactive delirium – Standard order
• Risperidone 0.25-0.5 mg PO bid PRN
• Haloperidol 0.5-1mg PO/IM q1h PRN severe agitation. Reassess after 3 doses.
• If patient has history of Parkinson's disease or Lewy Body Dementia:
• Seroquel 12.5mg PO bid PRN agitation. Lorazepam 0.5-1mg IM q1h PRN severe agitation. Reassess after 3 doses.

Conclusion

As the population ages, clinicians will encounter delirium more frequently as more patients have dementia and have multiple comorbidities. Prompt and efficient management of delirium is essential to preserve a patient's cognition and function, and of course, to decrease mortality.

Among non-delirious hospitalized patients who are at risk, prevention techniques such as the HELP (Hospital Elder Life Program) could reduce the incidence of delirium. One area of research also focuses on finding a delirium risk-prediction score. Hospital resources could then be used to provide prevention techniques targeting those patients who are at high risk of developing delirium, with the potential to decrease its sometimes-catastrophic consequences.

The clinical vignette revisited

Pre-operatively, this patient was already at high risk for delirium, due to her age, dementia, functional impairment and multiple comorbidities. Initial investigations mentioned above should be performed. The potential causes and management plan are summarized in the following table:

The non-pharmacological management of this patient includes removal of restraints, early mobilization, nutrition and speech-language pathology consult and promotion of night-time sleep.

Possible causes of patient's delirium	Management plan
Opioids (morphine)	Change to Dilaudid, and consider regular Dilaudid for 6-12 hours as delirious patients might not ask for pain medications
CHF exacerbation due to overhydration	Chest X-ray; increase Lasix if needed
Anemia due to blood loss	Follow Hb, transfuse if needed
Right lower extremity DVT	Venous Duplex
Worsening of Parkinson's disease due to Haldol and refusal to take Sinemet	Change Sinemet to equivalent dose per rectum Use Seroquel PO or Ativan IM for agitation if non-pharmacological approaches fail
Uncontrolled pain	Monitor and manage pain
Constipation	Mobilization, laxatives, DRE to R/O impaction
Urinary retention	PVR, in/out if needed
Stroke despite Coumadin bridging	Thorough neurological examination, CT/CTA head if high suspicion
Aspiration pneumonia due to Parkinsonism	Chest X-ray

FURTHER READING

1. Wise, M. G. (1986). Delirium. In R. E. Hales & S. C. Yudofsky (Eds.), American Psychiatric Press Textbook of Neuropsychiatry (pp. 89–103). Washington, DC: American Psychiatric Press Inc.

2. Marcantonio, E. R. Delirium in Hospitalized Older Adults. N Engl J Med 2017; 377:1456-1466. DOI: 10.1056/NEJMcp1605501

3. Chew, M.L. Anticholinergic activity of 107 medications commonly used by older adults. J Amer Geri Soc 2008; 56,7:1333-1341. DOI: 10.1111/j.1532-5415.2008.01737.

WHY DOES MY PATIENT HAVE GAIT & BALANCE DISORDERS?

Olivier Beauchet, MD, PhD, Professor of Geriatrics, Dr. Joseph Kaufmann Chair in Geriatric Medicine, Director of centre of excellence on aging and chronic diseases, McGill University,

Patient Scenario

An 87-year-old woman walks into your office unaided, without any noticeable gait abnormality. She reports that she has balance difficulties with fear of falling but denied any fall. The patient's medication list includes amlodipine 5 mg QD, metformin 500 mg BI, aspirin 80 md QD, atorvastatin 10 mg, donepezil 5 mg QD and temazepam as needed for sleep. Her body mass index is 18 kg/m². The daughter hands you an X-ray report indicating that the patient has severe osteoporosis, moderate spinal (cervical and lumbar) osteoarthritis associated with dorsal kyphosis.

Since your patient has a high risk of falls, you would like to determine the reason of balance complaints to decide whether she needs specific interventions.

Why is this question important?

Gait - the medical term used to describe the human locomotion - and balance disorders are prevalent in older individuals. It is difficult to ascertain prevalence as no accepted definition exists. However, it is estimated that at least 35 percent of individuals 65 and older report difficulty walking three city blocks or climbing one flight of stairs, and approximately 20 percent require the use of a mobility aid to ambulate. The prevalence of gait and balance disorders can reach 80 percent in the oldest-old (i.e., ≥ 85 years) individuals who live in residence.

Gait and balance characteristics change over the individual's lifetime with a decline of performance. Gait and balance disorders are usually defined as a decrease of performance (for instance, a slow gait speed) causing instability and falls. Gait and balance disorders are the most common cause of falls in individuals 65 and older. They are associated with an increased morbidity and mortality, disability, loss of independence, institutionalization and limited quality of life. Early identification and appropriate interventions may prevent gait and balance disorders and their related adverse consequences.

Which are the causes of gait and balance disorders?

Gait and balance disorders are usually multifactorial in origin and require a comprehensive assessment to determine contributing factors and targeted interventions. Most changes in gait and balance that occur in older individuals are related to physiological aging of the sensorimotor system combined with adverse consequences of chronic and acute medical conditions. The causes of gait and balance disorders fall under three categories of factors:

- The predisposing factors which are individually related and result from adverse consequences of physiological aging of the sensorimotor system combined with chronic medical conditions leading to chronic gait and balance instability.
- The precipitating factors which may be separated in two subtypes: those related to individual acute medical conditions and those related to physical activity inducing gait and balance instability.
- The environment combined with the physical activity while falling.

There is a complex synergic interaction between factors provoking gait and balance instability, explaining why gait and balance instability may fluctuate with time.

The main chronic medical conditions which affect gait and balance stability are:

- Visual impairment with abnormal distance vision including low visual acuity and low contrast sensitivity.
- Lower limb proprioception impairment.
- Lower limb poor muscle mass and strength.
- Lower limb joint deformity, podiatric abnormalities and back deformity (e.g.; kyphosis, scoliosis) related to osteoarthritis and osteoporosis.
- Obesity.
- Myelopathy.
- Normal-pressure hydrocephalus.
- Parkinson disease.
- Cerebellar dysfunction or degeneration.
- Vascular brain disease.
- Vestibular disorders.
- Cognitive impairment: from mild cognitive impairment to severe dementia.
- Depression.
- Fear of falling.

Any acute medical condition may increase gait and balance instability within hours and cause a motor deconditioning (i.e.; loss of body postural reflexes and inability to stand up and/or walk without assistance) in older individuals with predisposing factors to gait and balance disorders.

Who should be screened for gait and balance disorders?

- Adults aged 65 and over should be asked about or examined for gait and balance disorders at least once per year.
- Adults aged 65 and over who report a fall or have an acute medical condition should be asked about difficulties with gait and balance, and should be examined for gait and balance disorders.

What is the clinical assessment?

Clinical assessment should be separated into two main parts: global and analytic clinical assessment.
The global assessment detecting gait and balance difficulties begins with watching individuals as they rise from a chair or as they walk into the examination room. The use of a walking aide and its nature (i.e.; cane, walker, personal assistance and supervision) should be noticed and the individual should be asked about his/her subjective perception of gait and balance difficulties using a single question: "Do you have any difficulty walking?" with a graduated answer (i.e., never, almost never, sometimes, often, and very often).

This visual observation should be completed with three standardized motor tests providing an objective measure of gait and balance performance: The Timed up & Go (TUG) test, the five time to sit to stand test and the gait speed (distance divided by ambulation time) when walking a distance of 4 meters at a steady-state pace. The TUG measures in seconds the time it takes an individual to rise from a chair, walk a distance of 3 meters, turn, walk back to the chair and sit down. This test has been used extensively in geriatric medicine to examine balance, gait speed, and functional ability that would be required for the performance of basic activities of daily living in older people. A score ≥ 20 second should be considered as an abnormal performance. The Five-Times-Sit-to-Stand test (FTSS) measures in seconds the time it takes an individual to stand up from a chair five times as quickly as possible. This clinical test explores postural control and lower limb muscular strength. A score ≥ 15 seconds should be considered as an abnormal performance. Walking speed is a simple, objective, performance-based measure of lower limb neuromuscular function which not only allows detection of subtle impairments and preclinical diseases, but also is a sensitive marker of functional capacity in older adults. A gait speed at usual pace under 1 m/s should also be considered as abnormal.

The analytic clinical assessment includes collection of:

- Demographic (i.e., age in years and sex) and anthropometric items (height in meters [m], weight in kilograms [kg], body mass index (BMI) in kg/m^2), should be systematically assessed because each may influence gait and balance stability. In addition, the place of living should be considered as a binary variable home versus institution, and an institutionalized individual should be considered to have a higher risk of gait and balance disorders.

- Given that the burden of disease can influence gait and balance performance, it is important to assess this information as well. Different scales have been developed to score morbidity burden, but they remain difficult to use in clinical routine among older adults, especially because of possible recall bias in individuals with cognitive disorders, and lack of feasibility in daily practice. Medication data, including the number of drugs taken daily provides a global measure of morbidity status, and has been associated with physician-rated disease severity as well as with individual-rated health status. Hence, recording the use of drugs in the clinical assessment is required. Polypharmacy is defined as use of more than four different medications per day. The use of psychoactive drugs (i.e., benzodiazepines, antidepressants, neuroleptics), needs to be specially recorded.

- Information about falls, with a fall being defined as an event resulting in a person coming to rest unintentionally on the ground or at another lower level, not as the result of a major intrinsic event or an overwhelming hazard, in the previous 12 months period before the assessment, should be recorded. Information on recurrence (i.e.; >2 falls) and severity (defined as fractures, cranial trauma, large and/or deep skin lesion, post-fall syndrome (including an association of fear of falling (FOF), postural instability with absence of postural reflexes), inability to get up alone from ground, time on the ground > one hour, and hospitalization) are proposed for the data collection.

- FOF using the single question: "Are you afraid of falling?" with a graded answer (i.e., never, almost never, sometimes, often, and very often) should be asked to the patient as FOF is associated with a greater gait and/or balance instability.

- Collecting information on disorders or diseases that directly influence gait performance is also recommended. First, information on neurological disease (limited to the existence or non-existence of dementia) and other diseases (coded as yes or no) should be collected. Information on memory complaints, MCI, nature of dementia (i.e., Alzheimer Disease (AD), non-AD neurodegenerative, non-AD vascular, mixed), Parkinson disease, idiopathic normal pressure hydrocephalus, cerebellar disease, stroke, myelopathy and peripheral neuropathy should be recorded. A quantification of global cognitive functioning is also recommended, using for example The Mini Mental State Examination (/30) and The Montreal Cognitive Assessment (MoCA) if MMSE score is above 19/30.

- In addition, among the neuropsychiatric disorders, it is important to collect information about depression symptoms because they can lead to gait instability and falls. The 4-item geriatric depression scale should be used as a screening test. A measure of anxiety is also proposed using the 5-item Geriatric Anxiety Inventory.

- Information on major orthopaedic diagnoses (e.g., osteoarthritis) involving the lumbar vertebrae, pelvis or lower extremities, coded yes versus no, as well as the use of a walking aids, should also be recorded.

- Information on sensory and motor subsystems such as muscle strength, lower-limb proprioception and vision are required because the age-related impairment in the performance of these subsystems may affect gait performance.

First, the maximum isometric voluntary contraction (MVC) of hand grip strength must be measured with a hydraulic dynamometer. The test should be performed three times with the dominant hand. The mean value of MVC over the three trials should be used as the outcome measure. Second, distance binocular vision should be measured at a fixed distance with a standard scale. Vision needs to be assessed with corrective lenses if used regularly. Third, lower-limb proprioception should be evaluated with a graduated tuning fork placed on the tibial tuberosity measuring vibration threshold.

Is there a need for complementary investigations?

The role of laboratory testing and diagnostic evaluation for gait and balance disorders has not been well studied.

There is no systematic investigation recommended to perform. The following complementary investigations are recommended:

- Bone radiography in the event of acute pain, joint deformation and/or functional disability.
- Standard 12-lead ECG in case of dizziness.
- Blood glucose level in patients with diabetes.
- Serum 25OHD concentration if there is no vitamin D supplementation.

Cerebral imaging in the absence of specific indication based upon the clinical examination may not be necessary.

Which are the possible interventions?

It is recommended to suggest to the patient with gait and balance disorders, irrespective of the place of living, an intervention combining several of the following domaines:

- When possible, a revision of the medications to ascertain if the patient takes fall-related drugs (please see above) and/or the number of drugs is >5.
- The correction or the treatment of predisposing or modifiable precipitating factors (including environmental risk factors of falls);
- The wearing of shoes with broad, low heels (2 to 3 cm), and firm, thin soles with a high upper;
- The regular practice of walking and/or any other physical activity (the duration of exercise for prevention of recurrent falls remains unclear);
- A dietary calcium intake ranging from 1 to 1,5 gram per day;
- The use of an adapted walking aid;
- The correction of a potential vitamin D deficiency by a daily dose of at least 800IU.

It is recommended to prescribe physiotherapy, including:

- Working on static and dynamic postural balance;

- Increasing of the strength and muscular power of the lower limbs.
- Other techniques, including stimulation of sensory afferents or learning to stand up from the ground, may also be proposed.

Such interventions may involve rehabilitation professionals, such as occupational therapists. A regular physical activity should be performed at low to moderate intensity exercise. It is recommended to perform rehabilitation exercises with a professional, as well as between therapy sessions and after each session, in order to extend rehabilitation benefits to the daily life.

Scenario resolution

Your patient requires a specific gait and balance assessment as she is an oldest-old (i.e.; > 85 years) lady who reports balance difficulties.

Based on the information provided by the list of medications and the daughter, you can conclude that she has an objective gait and balance disorder caused by an accumulation of chronic medical conditions, which are:

- A polypharmacy: Six different medications are taken daily.
- A lower limb diabetic polyneuropathy causing proprioceptive impairment.

- An abnormal static posture due to spinal osteo-arthritis and osteoporosis deformaties
- A poor muscle mass and strength because of a malnutrition status (body mass index score 18 kg/m^2).
- A cognitive impairment due to a dementia because of the prescription of donepezil.

You can confirm you first analysis by performing a TUG test.

You can propose:

- To discontinue the temazepam,
- To continue anti-osteoporotic treatment and vitamin D supplementation.
- To a regular practice of walking and/or any other physical activity.

You can prescribe physiotherapy including:

- Working on static and dynamic postural balance.
- Increasing of the strength and muscular power of the lower limbs.

References

1. Nutt JG. Classification of gait and balance disorders. Adv Neurol 2001;87:135-141.

2. Seidler RD, Bernard JA, Burutolu TB, Fling BW, Gordon MT, Gwin JT, Kwak Y, Lipps DB. Motor control and aging: links to age-related brain structural, functional, and biochemical effects. Neurosci Biobehav Rev 2010;34:721-733.

3. Beauchet O, Dubost V, Revel Delhom C, Berrut G, Belmin J, French Society of Geriatrics and Gerontology. How to manage recurrent falls in clinical practice: guidelines of the French Society of Geriatrics and Gerontology. J Nutr Health Aging 2011; 15:79-84

4. Panel on Prevention of Falls in Older Persons, American Geriatrics Society and British Geriatrics Society. Summary of the Updated American Geriatrics Society/British Geriatrics Society clinical practice guideline for prevention of falls in older persons. J Am Geriatr Soc 2011; 59:148-157.

5. Salzman B. Gait and balance disorders in older adults. Am Fam Physician. 2010;82:61-68.

COULD MY PATIENT BE MALNOURISHED?

Jose A. Morais, MD, FRCP(C), Associate Professor and Director,
Division of Geriatric Medicine, McGill University, Associate Director,
Quebec Network for Research on Aging

Clinical vignette

An 82 year old widow has a 4.5 kg weight loss over the last 6 months following the death of her beloved husband. Her present BMI is 21 kg/m² and her triceps skinfold thickness is in the 10th percentile for age. She is known to have diabetes and osteoarthritis of both knees for which she uses a walker for indoor mobility. She denies being depressed, but her family physician prescribed a tricyclic antidepressant medication, soon after the death of her spouse. Since then, she complains of dry mouth with difficulty swallowing food and is constipated. Her other medications are metformin 850 mg BID and naprosyn 250 mg BID. The pertinent blood tests available disclosed an albumin of 38 g/L, CRP 2 mg/L, A1C 6%, creatinine 98 umol/L.

Since involuntary weight loss in older adults should always be taken seriously, there is a need to ascertain the presence of malnutrition, determine its risk factors, and propose a plan for assessment and management.

Why is malnutrition an important clinical problem?

Malnutrition is common in older people and in those who are frail and ill. In the healthy community-dwelling older person, its prevalence is about 2-5%, whereas in the frail, dependent elderly, it can reach 20-30%. In those living in nursing homes or in hospital, levels as high as 50-70% have been reported.

Malnutrition or more precisely, undernutrition, is a state of reduced food intake below recommended daily allowances that leads to loss of body mass (weight) and functional impairment. The functional deficiencies comprise physical performance such as grip strength and gait speed, immunocompetence and tissue repair capacity. As a consequence, malnourished older persons have higher risks of falls and fractures, delirium, depression, cognitive deficits, infections, hospitalisations with prolonged stay, decubitus ulcers and death.

Other terminologies are often used in conjunction with malnutrition. These are protein-energy malnutrition (PEM), anorexia, wasting, cachexia and sarcopenia. PEM refers to a global decrease in food intake with its health consequences and is equivalent to undernutrition/malnutrition; anorexia is a lack of appetite and wasting that is synonymous with loss of body mass. Wasting follows a lack of appetite without inflammation, and therefore, a preferential loss of adipose tissue over muscle mass is a predominant feature. Cachexia on the other hand is a catabolic condition often involving a high degree of inflammation from a disease such as cancer or congestive heart failure. Its prominent feature is suppression of appetite with proportionally more muscle loss than adipose tissue and with fatigue. Sarcopenia refers to a selective loss of muscle mass and strength associated with aging that has a large number of factors contributing to its development.

What are the risk factors for malnutrition?

Older adults are predisposed to anorexia due to intrinsic as well as exogenous causes. At the intrinsic physiological level, one needs to consider the adjustment of energy balance that occurs with aging. Aging is associated with loss of lean body mass, especially muscle mass, a metabolically active tissue, and therefore its loss leads to a decrease in the basal metabolic rate (energy spent at rest to maintain bodily functions). Furthermore, since there is also a progressive decline in physical activity, the total amount of energy ingested needs to be reduced, otherwise the elderly would gain considerable weight over time.

A theoretical model of anorexia of aging proposes a dysregulation of the appetite control center in the hypothalamus. This dysregulation is in part related to changes in brain neurotransmitters, such as NPY and dynorphin, the latter decreasing the pleasure associated with meals. It is also recognized that there is a higher circulating gastrointestinal peptide cholecystokinin (CCK) upon food ingestion, which is a potent central anorexigen. At the fundus of the stomach, there is reduced nitric oxide production with meals which contributes to a lesser relaxation of the stomach, therefore contributing to a precocious sensation of fullness. Older persons have also alterations in their taste perception from changes in the odor and taste capacities. Thirst perception is equally affected with age, which predisposes to dehydration.

Although the above factors are present with aging, they are not by themselves responsible for the decrease in food intake of older persons. Multiple other causes contribute as well. These include:

- Uncontrolled medical conditions that predispose to anorexia through the effect of inflammatory mediators (TNF-α and cytokines), pain, distress, lethargy, delirium, etc.
- Social-economic factors including isolation, poverty and institutionalization
- Masticatory and swallowing difficulties: e.g., poor fitting dentures and dysphagia

- Decrease in functional capacity caused by mobility problems, poor endurance and multiple co-morbidities, which affect the capability to purchase food and prepare meals
- Mental and cognitive disorders e.g., depression and dementia
- Peculiar habits such as aversion to certain foods and alcoholism
- Medications, in particular: digoxin, SSRIs, NSAIDs, metformin, antibiotics and psychoactive drugs

It is often difficult to distinguish a single factor as responsible in the vast majority of the cases, as more often several factors interact. The above pathological/physiological/environmental changes can be summarised in a mnemonic MEALS-ON-WHEELS, proposed by Morley EJ and Silver AJ Ann Intern Med 1995;123:850-9.

Below is an algorithm to assist in evaluating causes of PEM. In general it is helpful to determine if the patient is eating well despite losing weight. If it is the case, the patient is either suffering from malabsorption (a relatively easy diagnosis to make because of GI symptoms) or having increased needs for energy in conditions such as hyperthyroidism, diabetes, cancer, chronic infections or advanced COPD or CHF.

Factors Contributing to Malnutrition

MEALS ON WHEELS acronym helps to remember the common risk factors and causes of undernutrition in older adults

Medications (polypharmacy, herbal preparations)

Emotional causes (dysphoria, depression, psychosis)

Appetite disorders (anorexia tardive, abnormal eating attitudes)

Late-life paranoia (social isolation)

Swallowing disorders

Oral factors (tooth loss, periodontal infections, gingivitis, poorly fitting dentures)

No money (poverty)

Wandering (dementia)

Hyperactivity/hypermetabolism (tremors, movement disorders, thyrotoxicosis)

Enteral problems (chronic diarrhea, malabsorption syndromes)

Eating problems (altered food preferences, decreased taste and flavor perception)

Low-nutrient diets (low-salt, low-cholesterol, antidiabetic, fad diets)

Shopping and food-preparation problems (impaired mobility, unsafe environment, inadequate transportation)

On the other hand, if the patient is not eating well, then a first step is to verify accessibility to food (poverty, mobility issues and meal preparation). If these are not factors, then consider masticatory and swallowing difficulties. If these are not an issue, it is likely that we are facing a case of anorexia from medications, depression, dementia or multi-morbidity.

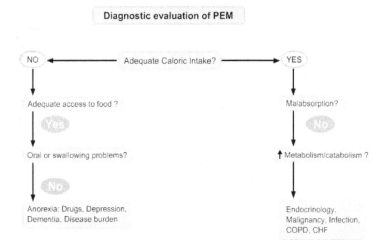

How is the diagnosis of malnutrition made?

On history taking, one reliable but often-ignored parameter of malnutrition is weight loss. A history of 5-10 % weight loss over 6 months (> 3 kg) or 2-3% in 1-2 months, is a significant amount that threatens the general health. Changes in food habits for any reason (difficulty swallowing, poverty) and GI symptoms (nausea, abdominal cramps, and diarrhea) are other important items of information. Any new drugs being prescribed? Typically, one eats three meals a day and eating less frequently puts one at risk. Food assessment is done by a registered dietician through different of dietary intake assessment methods, each with its own limitations.

<u>On physical examination</u>, in addition to a low weight for height or a low body mass index (BMI) < 22 kg/m², signs of ascites/edema or decreased skin turgor are suggestive of malnutrition. Loss of typical roundness of the face, shoulder and buttocks is often encountered as well as muscle loss at the temporal areas, biceps, thigh and calf. Specific vitamin deficiencies leading to angular stomatitis of the mouth and glossitis are late signs. All of these signs become more difficult to assess in the elderly due to lack of specificity and sensitivity. For example, a decrease in skin elasticity with aging and other causes such as venous stasis contribute to peripheral edema. Typically, it is the dietitian who carries out the relevant anthropometric measurements (body and limb circumferences and skinfold thickness). Values below the 15th percentile for sex and age are very suggestive of malnutrition. Physical performance tests such as handgrip strength using a dynamometer may corroborate the diagnosis.

<u>At the laboratory level</u>, the serum albumin level is the most useful parameter. This protein is produced by the hepatocytes when adequate amino acids and energy are available. The total body albumin pool is about 300 g with 1/3 lying in the interstitial space and its half-life is 20 days. The albumin value doesn't need to be at 35 g/L to be considered low. Any value below 40 g/L puts the patient at risk, although typically values < 38 g/L are used as cut-off for malnutrition. If coupled with a low cholesterol value of

< 4 mmol/L, the likelihood of malnutrition is greatly augmented. Despite adequate dietary intake of both energy and protein, albumin and pre-albumin are decreased in 1) the presence of inflammation (cancer, immunological disorders, trauma, and infections), 2) patients who have received large amounts of intravenous fluids (dilutional), 3) protein losing enteropathies (losses through the gut) or 4) nephropathies (losses through the kidney). On the other hand, albumin in the interstitial space can be recruited to the circulation during periods of poor intake without inflammation, which is the case in simple anorexia (wasting).

Measurement of pre-albumin values is rarely required, since it is under the same regulatory control as albumin. It may however be useful in monitoring the response to a nutritional intervention due to its half-life of 2 days. Cut-off values for undernutrition are below 180 mg/L.

Low hemoglobin and lymphocyte counts are less specific and are a late manifestation of malnutrition. In the absence of any other cause, a lymphocyte count below 800 cells/mL is however a sign of severe malnutrition. Anergy testing is rarely performed but would likely demonstrate a reduced immune response.

Useful tools for the diagnosis of malnutrition

There is no single parameter with the requisite sensitivity and specificity; thus, it is recommended that a combination of 3 or 4 indices from different domains (history, physical examination and investigation) be assessed. In this regard, several screening and diagnostic tools are available. Among these, two have received significant attention, the Mini Nutritional Assessment (MNA) and the Subjective Global Assessment (SGA).

The MNA has been validated in many settings, including long term care and acute care hospital sites and can be used to screen and diagnose early undernutrition in frail persons. It comprises items that are related to cognition, mental and physical function as well as dietary intake and anthropometric measurements. The total possible score is 30--values below 17 are diagnostic of malnutrition, between 17-24 suggest a risk of malnutrition and above 24, signify good nutritional status. A shorter version based on the first 14 points of the MNA exists that is almost as reliable as the full version for screening and has the merit of precluding a full assessment if values are 12 or higher. If score of the shorter version is < 11, one should perform the full MNA. The MNA formula can be downloaded at no cost: http://www.mna-elderly.com/mna_forms.html

The SGA is a clinical assessment of nutrition status based on history and physical examination. In taking a history, one reviews changes in dietary intake, weight loss, GI symptoms and functional capacity and on physical examination, one should look for signs of undernutrition, including ascites and edema. It requires only minimal training. The rater then classifies patients subjectively as well-nourished, mildly/

moderately malnourished or severely malnourished. This tool has been validated with respect to clinical outcomes and has a good inter-observer agreement. The form can be downloaded at no cost: http://nutritioncareincanada.ca/

What are the interventions to reverse malnutrition?

Before proposing an intervention, it is necessary to determine the factors contributing to undernutrition in the specific case instance (review the mnemonic MEALS-ON-WHEELS). Intervention can be as broad as helping with meal preparation, providing spoon feeding or diagnosing an underlying medical condition.

The first step in the management of undernutrition consists in identifying and treating the underlying causative factors. If the nutrition status does not show improvement in 1 week with this first-line approach, than nutritional support may be necessary. If not done previously, it is recommended at this stage to seek the advice of a dietician. Below is an algorithm with an approach to treatment of malnutrition.

The dietician will assess in detail the patient's food intake and preferences and will propose a meal plan with more frequent meals and snacks enriched with food additives to enhance energy intake to 30-40 kcal/kg/d and protein to 1.2 - 1.5 g/kg/d. If this doesn't suffice, an oral formula supplement can be offered together with food additives. It is best to provide such added formula feedings in the evening to avoid interference with meals resulting in meal replacement without higher total energy intakes. A high density formula supplement of 1.5 - 2 calories/mL can deliver up to 400 calories with as much as 15 g of protein per container.

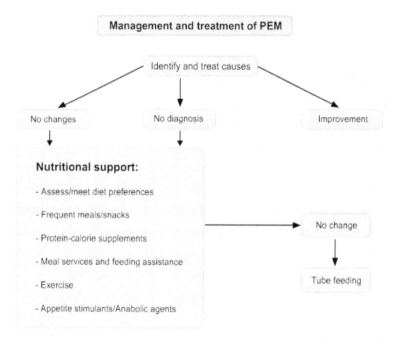

Whenever possible, combining some degree of physical activity such as frequent short walks with the dietary intervention can ameliorate appetite and food intake. The use of oral orexigenic medications is controversial in older adults, including the new synthetic tetrahydrocannabinol molecule, dronabinol. However, in case of depression, one should consider mirtazapine, a tetracyclic antidepressant with appetite stimulating properties. Hormones are useful only in those in whom a deficiency state has been diagnosed,

In cases in which malnutrition progresses rapidly, assessment in an acute care setting may be considered to provide access to the different specialists, investigational platforms and interdisciplinary teams. In certain cases, enteral feeding may be indicated and can be initiated.

Resolution of the clinical vignette

The higher the number of indices of malnutrition, the greater the certainty of its presence. In the case of the person described at the outset of this chapter, the weight loss of more than 3 kg in 6 months, a BMI of less than 22 kg/m^2 and the low triceps skinfold percentile are very suggestive.

The risk factors comprise isolation (death of husband), recent bereavement, side effects from the medication (dry mouth, constipation), swallowing difficulties, chronic pains from arthritis and reduced mobility to purchase food. Consideration should include metformin due to its propensity to suppress appetite and naprosyn which can lead to peptic ulcer disease (nausea).

Serum albumin is often used as one of the criteria to diagnose malnutrition. In the present case, a value of 38 g/L can be misleading since there is mild dehydration (Cr 98 umol/L), that may be responsible for a factitious elevation.

Since CRP is in the normal range, it rules out inflammation. The A1C level is also too low for this frail patient suggesting overly 'tight' control of capillary glucose putting the patient at risk of hypoglycemia.

The amount of weight loss indicates referral to a dietitian, but at this stage, one can emphasise the avoidance of food restriction or a severe diabetic diet, which is often the case in diabetic patients. The dietitian is likely to suggest high density food additives with regular meals and snacks as a first approach. If no change in weight is observed at follow-up in 2 weeks' time, an oral formula supplement should be provided for evening consumption, to avoid interference with regular meals, thus resulting in little gain in total daily calorie intake.

A medication review is mandatory. Metformin should be reduced to 250 mg po BID and Naprosyn discontinued. For pain management, one can offer acetaminophen. The tricyclic antidepressant should be stopped and clinical review after 2 weeks can ascertain if symptoms of dry mouth, swallowing difficulties and constipation have disappeared. If not, one would need to consider a GI assessment.

Finally, a functional evaluation should be undertaken and community support offered to this patient to compensate and support her life situation. Above all, we should help overcome her isolation and assess her meal preparation and food purchasing capacities.

References

1. Kucukerdonmez O, Navruz Varli S, Koksal E. Comparison of Nutritional Status in the Elderly According to Living Situations. J Nutr Health Aging. 2017;21(1):25-30.
2. Landi F Calvani R, Tosato M et al. Anorexia of Aging: Risk Factors, Consequences, and Potential Treatments. Nutrients 2016, 8, 69; doi:10.3390/nu8020069
3. Stajkovic S[1], Aitken EM, Holroyd-Leduc J. Unintentional weight loss in older adults. CMAJ. 2011 Mar 8;183(4):443-9. doi: 10.1503/cmaj.101471
4. Pirlich M, Lochs H. Nutrition in the elderly. Best Practice & Res Clin Gastroenterol. 2001; 15: 869-884
5. Gaddey H L., Holder K. Unintentional Weight Loss in Older Adults. Am Fam Physician. 2014;89:718-722

INCONTINENCE IN OLDER ADULTS

Samer Shamout MD, MSc., Fellow, Division of Urology, McGill University
Lysanne Campeau, MDCM, PhD, FRCS(C)),
Assistant Professor of Surgery, Division of Urology, McGill University
Division of Urology, Department of Surgery, Jewish General Hospital,
McGill University, Montreal, Quebec, Canada

Clinical vignette

An 83-year-old man with Alzheimer disease is being cared for at home. During the past 2 months, his wife has noticed that it is increasingly difficult for him to make it to the restroom in time to urinate. He has stopped telling her when he needs to use the restroom, and she is unable to direct him to the restroom in the house quick enough. This is causing significant caregiver stress. His wife believes his cognition has begun to worsen during the past 6 months, and she is considering placing him in a nursing home. His medication list includes terazosin 2 mg at bedtime, aspirin 81 mg daily, donepezil 10 mg at bedtime, lisinopril 5 mg daily, and venlafaxine extended release 75 mg daily. His Mini-Mental State Examination score is 15/30, and his Geriatric Depression Scale is 3/15. Standing blood pressure is 110/70 mm Hg.

The urinary incontinence is a significant problem for this patient and his caregiver, and should be addressed with appropriate workup and management plan.

Why is urinary incontinence a remarkable clinical condition in elderly population?

Urinary incontinence (UI), is a common and undertreated condition of morbidity in Canada and worldwide, with peak prevalence in the geriatric population. Approximately, 3.3 million (10%) Canadians experience urinary incontinence, of whom 30 to 60% are over 65 years old. The prevalence of incontinence increases noticeably with age, affecting 19% of women and 10% of men above 60 years old. Urinary incontinence (UI), is defined as the complaint of involuntary leakage of urine.

The cost of UI in this population extends beyond monetary costs. It has a substantial negative impact on physical, psychological and health related quality of life. Moreover, UI has a great economic burden on society and on the healthcare system. It has been linked to many other critical health risks, including increased risk of hospitalization, frailty, fractures, functional disability and depression. The social implications of incontinence include diminished self-esteem, restriction of social and sexual activities and increased caregiver burden.

Unfortunately, elderly individuals encounter several obstacles in obtaining treatment for their problems. UI is rarely discussed by patients, many of whom are less likely to seek healthcare for this condition as they assume that UI is a part of aging process and there is no existing successful treatment.

What are the risk factors for UI?

The etiology of UI among the geriatric population is different and often multifactorial. As people age, physiological and functional changes in the lower urinary tract may contribute to the loss of continence in this population. Frail elderly people may have multiple comorbid medical illnesses, lifestyle, and medication changes that can cause or predispose to UI. Therefore, the evaluation and management of UI in older adults should be multidisciplinary with comprehensive understanding of the multidimensional concept of continence.

Risk factors for UI in women include changes related to anatomy, previous childbirth, hysterectomy, and menopause. Loss of estrogen at menopause and changes in the pelvic connective tissue support may explain higher prevalence of UI in postmenopausal women. On the other side, factors associated with UI in men include prostatic enlargement or prostate surgery. Despite surgical advances, UI is frequently observed following prostate surgery, with reported estimates ranging from 6% to nearly 70%.

Multiple other conditions are also associated with UI in the frail elderly population. These include:

- Uncontrolled comorbid medical conditions that predispose to polyuria or increased nighttime urine production (e.g., congestive heart failure, peripheral venous insufficiency, diabetes mellitus, sleep apnea)
- Conditions resulting in impaired mobility and/or cognition (e.g., stroke, Parkinson's disease, degenerative joint disease, dementia)
- Constipation and fecal impaction that may contribute to double incontinence (urinary and fecal)
- Mental and cognitive disorders e.g., depression and dementia
- Medications: diuretics, calcium channel blockers, prostaglandin inhibitors, alpha-adrenoceptor blockers, selective serotonin reuptake inhibitors, cholinesterase inhibitors, opioid analgesics, psychotropic drugs and systemic hormone replacement therapy.
- Environmental factors e.g., inaccessible toilets or unavailable caregivers for toileting assistance.

In general, it is challenging to distinguish a single etiology responsible in the vast majority of geriatric population, as more often several factors interact. The above possible causes of reversible UI can be summarised in a mnemonic DIAPPERS (Delirium, Infection, Atrophic vaginitis, Psychological, Pharmacologic, Excess urine output, Restricted mobility and Stool impaction).

How is the diagnosis of UI made?

There are different types of UI in elderly population: urgency urinary incontinence (UUI) (involuntary loss of urine associated with urgency), stress urinary incontinence SUI (involuntary loss of urine on effort or physical exertion, or on sneezing/coughing), and mixed UI (a combination of SUI and UUI). A concomitant related condition which is associated with UUI is called overactive bladder syndrome (OAB), defined as urinary urgency, usually accompanied by frequency and nocturia, with or without urgency UI, in the absence of urinary tract infection or other obvious pathology. Other distinct entities are nocturia (frequent nocturnal micturition), and 'functional' incontinence (incontinence caused by either physical or cognitive impairment, with no identifiable lower urinary tract disorder), all being associated with extensive patient and caregiver burden.

Table 1: Common types of Urinary Incontinence				
Overactive bladder	Stress UI	Mixed UI	Impaired Bladder Emptying	Functional incontinence
Urinary urgency, with or without urgency incontinence often with urinary frequency and nocturia	Urinary loss in association with exertion such as coughing, laughing or lifting	Symptoms of both urgency incontinence and exertional incontinence (take a careful history as urgency or precipitancy is often reported by women with stress UI only)	Incomplete emptying is not well reported by men, but more so by women. A large post-void residual volume without symptoms (recurrent UTI, frequency, dribble, upper tract involvement) does not need treatment (a 250-ml residual volume may be acceptable in older people)	Incontinence unrelated to an underlying disorder or lower urinary tract function, perhaps related to either physical or cognitive impairment
Modified from Urinary incontinence in older adults. *Medicine*. 2017;45(1):23-27.				

How should patients be investigated ?
(see appendix for grading)

Unlike urinary incontinence evaluation in younger adults, frail older persons often require a comprehensive approach. The basic evaluation should primarily emphasize identification of transient and established causes of UI, assess the patient's environment and existing support, the degree of bother to the patient, and recognize other less common but serious entities that may trigger incontinence. The primary step is active screening for UI in the geriatric population, as more than 50% of elderly patients do not report their urinary symptoms to their health care providers. This could be due to numerous reasons, including social embarrassment, coping with symptoms, or misunderstanding that UI is a part of aging process and nothing can be done to improve this condition **(grade A)**. The patient history is often the most important element in recognizing the type, severity, and burden of incontinence for those patients. Commonly, clinical evaluation requires numerous office visits for frail older individuals in order to perform the necessary tests and to avoid additional assessment in patients who respond to ordinary measures.

History

The history should identify treatable, potentially reversible comorbid conditions, functional and cognitive impairment, and current medications that can cause or exacerbate UI in frail older people **(grade B)**. The mnemonic DIAPPERS has been commonly utilized to remember these conditions. The basic assessment must include an evaluation of the frequency and duration of symptoms, associated factors or events, precipitating and influential factors, and any measures of control that have already been used. During the history, account should be taken of the patient's medical and surgical history (ie, bowel, menstrual, obstetric, and sexual history), and risk factors which helps recognize possible influencing factors on symptoms. Furthermore, fluid/volume status, symptom severity, accessibility to toilets and social support, patient's and caregivers' expectations for UI care, should be explicitly explored **(grade B)**. It is also essential to consider the patient's likely level of cooperation, overall prognosis and life expectancy **(grade C)**.

In frail elderly people with bothersome nocturia, the treating physician should focus on detecting any potential triggering factors, including sleep apnea, nocturnal polyuria, and conditions associated with elevated post void residual (PVR). A complete and precise bladder diary (frequency-volume chart) of a minimum 3 days' duration can be a useful tool in the assessment of individuals with nocturia **(grade C)**. However, this may not always be feasible for all patients and caregivers.

Physical examination

The initial step is to perform a relevant pelvic or genital and rectal examination to evaluate for vaginal\genital atrophy, pelvic organ prolapse, prostate nodules or masses, sphincter tone, faecal impaction and the presence of a distended bladder or a pelvic mass. The initial physical examination should also include cognitive and functional assessments as well as examination for relevant neurological conditions (e.g. Parkinson's disease, stroke, spinal stenosis, and cauda equina syndrome) to rule out potential comorbid illnesses, which can directly influence continence status.

TABLE 2: Recommendation for initial evaluation of older adults with urinary incontinence*
Recommendations
Assess, treat and re-assess potentially treatable conditions (DIAPPERS)
Medical History
Evaluate treatment expectations regarding the continence paradigm
Physical examination including cognition, functional assessment, neurological and rectal examinations
Urine analysis
* Modified from 2012 update: guidelines for adult urinary incontinence collaborative consensus document for the canadian urological association. Can Urol Assoc J. 2012;6(5):354-363.

Useful tools for the diagnosis of UI

Basic investigations

- Dipstick urinalysis is recommended as an initial UI assessment, it helps to identify urinary tract infections as well as other abnormalities such as hematuria, pyuria, and/or bacteruria. All patients should be screened for haematuria **(grade C)**, while persistent pattern should prompt further evaluation, including upper tract imaging and cystoscopy.

- Measurement of the post-void residual volume is considered fundamental to an initial UI assessment to investigate for incomplete bladder emptying in frail older patients with long standing diabetes mellitus, previous history of urinary retention, recurrent urinary tract infections, medications known to decrease detrusor contractility (e.g., anticholinergics), severe constipation, complex neurologic disease, as well as persistent or deteriorating UI despite treatment **(grade C)**.
- Bladder diaries recording details of fluid intake, voiding times, and volumes are an appropriate assessment tool which help determine UI type, severity, and circumstances. A minimum of three days diary is recommended.
- Serum electrolytes, creatinine, and glucose maybe required if there is concern for renal impairment or in older adults with polyuria.

Specialist investigation

- Routine multichannel urodynamics testing is not necessary, but possibly warranted when diagnostic uncertainty may impact treatment decision, in patients who have not experienced significant improvement in symptoms despite prior therapy, and for patients considering invasive treatment.

Urodynamic evaluation in frail older persons is safe, feasible, and reproducible.

- More invasive investigation such as cystoure-throscopy is a potential diagnostic tool used in outpatient urology settings, indicated in the presence of hematuria or otherwise unexplained pelvic pain.

What are the interventions to reverse UI?

Before recommending a therapeutic intervention, it is crucial to determine the factors contributing to UI in the specific case presentation (review the mnemonic DIAPPERS). In the frail elderly patient, initial management is based first on the precise diagnosis of the type of UI experienced by the patient, severity of symptoms and bother, expectations and concerns of the patient and their caregiver(s). Treatment preferences, the level of cooperation, and the overall prognosis and life expectancy should also be considered. Below is an algorithm with an approach to treatment of UI.

Modified from 2012 update: guidelines for adult urinary incontinence collaborative consensus document for the Canadian Urological Association. *Can Urol Assoc J.* 2012;6(5):354-363.

Abbreviation: UI: urinary incontinence; BOO: bladder outlet obstruction; DHIC: detrusor hyperactivity with impaired contractility; UTI: urinary tract infection; CIC: clean intermittent catheterization.

Conservative and behavioral treatment strategies are useful in the broad management of UI **(grade C)**. lifestyle modifications and behavioral interventions that may be helpful include:

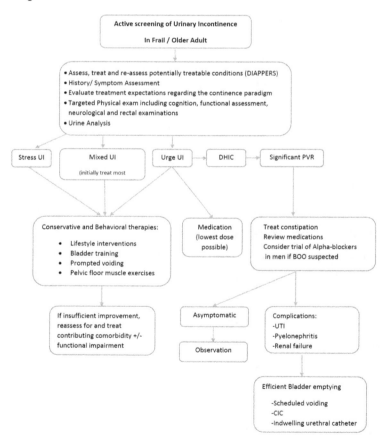

- Avoiding excess fluid intake, caffeinated drinks, and alcohol.
- Weight loss has been shown to be beneficial in reducing UI in morbidly obese women.
- Bladder training for capable patients and prompt voiding for frail and cognitively impaired individuals **(grade B)**.
- Pelvic muscle exercises may be considered, but evidence on their effectiveness are deficient **(grade C)**.
- Adjunctive management considerations for the geriatric population involve appropriate continence products and devices, along with proper skin hygiene and breakdown prevention of the external genitalia, and perineum.

Pharmacotherapy does not cure UI, but is often considered for symptomatic relief particularly in UUI. In the elderly population, any drug treatment should be started very carefully due to several factors, which include: polypharmacy, drug-drug interactions, impact on cognitive function, high potential for adverse events in this patient population. Additionally, it should be started with a low dose regimen and titrated gradually with regular assessment of clinical benefits and side effects. Table 3 summarizes recommendations for pharmacologic therapy in the geriatric population with urinary incontinence.

TABLE 3: Summary of Age-related pharmacokinetics changes, and their potential effect on urinary incontinence drugs

Parameter	Age-related changes	Potentially Affected UI Medications
Absorption	Minimal quantitative change despite delayed gastric emptying	Extended-release formulations
	Decrease subcutaneous fat	Topical preparations
Distribution	Decrease in lean body mass leads to: -Longer half-life of lipophilic agents -Higher serum concentration of hydrophilic agents	Tricyclic antidepressants
	low protein binding in older adults with low albumin level, give rise to greater concentration of free drug molecules	Tolterodine
Metabolism (hepatic)	Decreased oxidation/reduction reactions No change in hepatic glycosylation	Tricyclic antidepressants
	Decreased Hepatic blood flow and hepatic mass: less first-pass effect and increased serum level of un-metabolized drug	Oxybutynin, tolterodine, solifenacin, darifenacin
	Stereoselective selectivity in metabolism (hypothetical)	Enantiomers
	Cytochrome P450	Oxybutynin, tolterodine, solifenacin, darifenacin, mirabegron, 5-hydroxymethyl tolterodine
Excretion (renal)	Decrease in renal clearance (⁻GFR)	Tolterodine, fesoterodine

Modified from "CUA guideline on adult overactive bladder." *Canadian Urological Association Journal* 11.5 (2017): E142.
Abbreviation: GFR = glomerular filtration rate

These interventions should be individually tailored; and in certain patients a combination of the above approaches may be utilized. However, compliance may be a concern with some forms of therapy. Ultimately, consideration of specialist referral is recommended for older adults with hematuria, pelvic pain, complex neurologic disease, prior pelvic surgery, and a response to initial management that is insufficient. Identifying incontinence is the most important step. Nowadays, various therapeutic interventions are available for this prevalent geriatric problem, but the first priority should be directed to encourage elderly people to discuss their urinary symptoms with health care provider(s).

Many older people will require continence products (pads and protective garments). However, these products should be offered following a proper assessment and management plan or as a short-term relief until definitive diagnosis is explored. Indwelling urethral catheters or intermittent catheterization may be necessary for older adults with a significant PVR and impaired bladder emptying. It should be reserved when medical or surgical treatment is not possible and should not be considered as a replacement approach for nursing care of older adults with incontinence.

Summary
UI is a highly prevalent condition in the geriatric population and is associated with considerable patient, caregiver, and healthcare system burden. It represents a geriatric

condition with multiple risk factors and modifiers that include age-related changes, potentially comorbid conditions, medications, and functional impairments. Active screening for UI among frail older people is strongly recommended. A comprehensive initial evaluation requires assessment of potentially reversible conditions and impairments, as well as detailed history, physical exam, and urinalysis.

UI management in this population involves a multidisciplinary and stepwise approach progressing from lifestyle and behavioral modifications, pharmacotherapy to more invasive treatment strategies, as needed.

Appendix a- Grade of recommendation·	
Grade	Nature of recommendations
A	Based on clinical studies of good quality and consistency addressing the specific recommendations and including at least one randomised trial
B	Based on well-conducted clinical studies but without randomised clinical trials
C	Made despite the absence of directly applicable clinical studies of good quality
D	Evidence inconsistent/inconclusive (no recommendation possible) or the evidence indicates that the drug should not be recommended
* Modified from 2012 update: guidelines for adult urinary incontinence collaborative consensus document for the canadian urological association. Can Urol Assoc J. 2012;6(5):354-363.	

References[1-6]

1. Bettez M, Tu le M, Carlson K, et al. 2012 update: guidelines for adult urinary incontinence collaborative consensus document for the canadian urological association. *Can Urol Assoc J.* 2012; 6 (5): 354-363.

2. Thuroff JW, Abrams P, Andersson KE, et al. EAU guidelines on urinary incontinence. *Eur Urol.* 2011; 59 (3): 387-400.

3. Shaw C, Wagg A. Urinary incontinence in older adults. *Medicine.* 2017; 45 (1): 23-27.

4. Searcy JAR. Geriatric Urinary Incontinence. *Nurs Clin North Am.* 2017; 52 (3): 447-455.

5. Weiss BD. Diagnostic evaluation of urinary incontinence in geriatric patients. *American family physician.* 1998; 57: 2675-2694.

6. Corcos J, Przydacz M, Campeau L, et al. CUA guideline on adult overactive bladder. *Canadian Urological Association Journal.* 2017; 11(5): E142.

POLYPHARMACY AND DEPRESCRIBING IN THE ELDERLY

Louise Mallet, B.Sc.Pharm., Pharm.D., BCGP, FESCP, FOPQ
Professor in clinical pharmacy, Faculty of Pharmacy,
University of Montreal
Pharmacist in geriatrics, McGill University Health Center, Glen site
E-mail: louise.mallet@umontreal.ca

Clinical vignette

Mrs. D is a 92-year-old woman who lives alone in an upper duplex. She sustained a fall last week. She has two daughters that are involved in her care and visit their mother at least twice a week. Mrs. D needs help with ADLs (Activities of Daily Living) such as washing. She receives private help once a week for bathing. She also has a cleaning person who comes once a week. She still cooks but her daughters bring her meals that can be heated in the microwave. She dresses by herself and goes out with friends twice a month. It is mentioned by the daughters that Mrs. D does not always take her medications as prescribed. They often find pills on the floor when they visit. There are no known allergies

Past medical history is significant for hypertension, diabetes type 2, hypothyroidism, dyslipidemia, insomnia, constipation and a history of falls.

Weight: 50 kg. Height: 165 cm. Patient says she lost 5 kg in past 3 months.

Laboratory results from a week ago disclose (normal values in parenthesis):

- Na: 129 mmol/L (133-143)
- K: 4.4 mmol/L (3.5-5.0)
- Mg: 0.60 mmol/L (0.75-1.25)
- Creatinine: 85 μmol/L (40-85; stable)
- Albumin: 39 g/L (8-50)
- TSH: 9 μU/mL (04-4.4)
- Vitamin B12: 176 pmol/L (> 133)
- HbA1c 6,5% (4.3-6)
- Calculated Cr Cl using Cockcroft/Gault formula: 30 mL/min (>60)
- Blood glucose reported by daughter: between 4 and 7 mmol/L (3.9-11; done once a week at different times during the week)

Her current medication list is as follows:

- Amlodipine 5 mg po daily

- Pantoprazole 40 mg po daily
- Furosemide 40 mg po daily
- Levothyroxine 88 mcg po daily
- Metformin 850 mg po bid
- Atorvastatin 40 mg po daily
- Glyburide 5 mg po bid
- Docusate sodium 100 mg po bid
- Citalopram 20 mg po daily for the past 10 years
- Lorazepam 1 mg po at bedtime, prn
- Acetaminophen (Tylenol PM^MD) 1 tablet po at bedtime, prn

Her medications are delivered in vials. She has her own system to organize her medications. She prepares her medications for one week at a time using vials.

This case illustrates the problems with polypharmacy in older patients. This chapter will present a systematic process to optimize the medications prescribed for Mrs. D.

« *When an elderly patient presents with a status change, unless proven otherwise, it should be assumed to be a medication related problem* ».

Jerry Gurwitz M.D.

What is polypharmacy?

Polypharmacy is common in the elderly. However, there is no standard definition for polypharmacy. The World Health Organization (WHO) defines polypharmacy as multiple medicines for chronic use at the same time, usually more than 4 medications. Some authors have defined polypharmacy as "the prescription of more medications than clinically indicated, use of unnecessary drug, use of ineffective medication, the presence of therapeutic duplications or the concurrent use of 2 to 9 different therapeutic agents. Excessive polypharmacy is defined as the concurrent use of at least 10 medications in older adults.

Polypharmacy has been associated with decreased physical and social functioning, increased risk of falls, delirium, decreased adherence to medication, higher costs, emergency room visits, hospital admissions, nursing home placement and death.

In Canada, 20% percent of older adults aged 65 to 74 take 10 medications or more per day. This percentage increases to 32% for those aged 75 to 84 and to 40% for those≥ 85 years of age. It is reported that 30% of hospitalization in older adults 75 years of age and over are related to medications. (Canadian Institute for Health Information *2014*)

What is deprescribing?

Deprescribing is the process of stopping an inappropriate medication, supervised by a health care professional with the goal of managing polypharmacy and improving outcomes. Inappropriate medications are defined as medications in which risks outweigh benefits. Patient's goals, life expectancy, values, preferences and level of care should be discussed in the context of deprescribing. The activity of deprescribing should be part of the continuum of prescribing. It is a patient-centered intervention which includes patient consent, and close monitoring. Deprescribing encompasses the process of deciding with the patient which medications can be discontinued, planning a cessation protocol when needed and monitoring the plan and follow-up.

Which factors should be considered when evaluating medications in the elderly?

Is the patient really taking the medication?

- Ask the patient to bring medications (prescribed, over the counter, vitamins, eye drops, natural products, essential oils etc.). Mrs. D has a bottle of Tylenol PM[MD] which contains Acetaminophen 500 mg and diphenhydramine 25 mg. Diphenhydramine is an anticholinergic medication which can have an impact on her cognition and also cause falls. She has a history of falls and sustained a fall last week. She says that she recently bought this product as suggested by a friend. She took it once and did not like the feeling of it.

- TSH is elevated. Is Mrs. D taking her levothyroxine correctly? Daughter says that pills are found on the floor on a regular basis when she visits. It is suggested to continue the same dose of levothyroxine for now and repeat TSH in one month.

- Verify which system is used to help take her medication; dispill, dosett or other self-created system. Ask Mrs. D what she does when she forgets to take her medications. Verify with the community pharmacist whether she renews her medication on a regular basis. For example, Mrs. D has a prescription for lorazepam, a benzodiazepine, prescribed "prn" or as needed for sleep. It is important to verify if she takes it every night on a regular basis or say, once a week to avoid the risk of precipitating withdrawal symptoms. Benzodiazepines have been shown to increase the risk of falls, hip fractures, cognitive impairment, delirium, dementia and traffic accidents.

- Ask Mrs D if she knows the indication for each her medications; is she taking all her prescribed medications on a regular basis and if not, the reasons why (side effects, too many medications or forgetting to take them).

What are the current indications for each drug?

- Verify the indication for each medication.
- Verify the presence of a medication cascade. A prescribing cascade is observed when an adverse drug reaction is misinterpreted as a new medical problem. A second medication is prescribed which places the patient at risk of adverse drug reaction or potential drug-drug interactions. This domino effect can go on if not recognized by the health care provider. Some examples of prescribing cascades can be found below.
- Consider discontinuation or tapering the medication if no valid indication.
- Match each medication with a medical problem. For Mrs. D:

Examples of prescribing cascade		
Furosemide	→	urinary incontinence → oxybutynin
Amlodipine	→	peripheral edema → furosemide
Risperidone	→	rigidity → levodopa + carbidopa
Ciprofloxacin	→	hallucination → risperidone
Atorvastatin	→	leg pains → quinine
Digoxin	→	nausea/vomiting → metoclopramide
Venlafaxine	→	hyponatremia → salt supplements

Medications	Medical problems
Amlodipine	Hypertension
Furosemide	Lower leg edema from use of amlodipine? Medication cascade?
Atorvastatin	Hypercholesterolemia ?
Metformin Glyburide	Diabetes
Pantoprazole	GI problems?
Levothyroxine	Hypothyroidism
Docusate Sodium	Constipation
Insomnia	Lorazepam, Tylenol PM^MD
Citalopram	Depression?

What is Mrs. D's life expectancy and what are her expectations and preferences?

- Discuss with Mrs. D her expectations and preferences in terms of her medications.
- Estimate Mrs. D's life expectancy and objectives of treatment. She has a limited life expectancy between 1,9 and 3,9 years based on published literature.
- Define the therapeutic objective for the use of atorvastatin for Mrs. D. Suggest to discontinue considering her age.
- If a new medication is added, verify the time for benefit before prescribing considering her limited life expectancy.

- Identify medications which may cause harm. For example, use the American Geriatrics Society (AGS) Beers Criteria for potentially inappropriate medication (PIM) use in older adults, to verify which medications are potentially inappropriate.

AGS Beers Criteria for PIM	Reasons
Glyburide	Severe hypoglycemia
Citalopram	Hyponatremia, falls
Lorazepam	Slowness, confusion, falls
Pantoprazole	Use > 8 weeks causes hypomagnesemia, risk of Clostridium difficile infection

Considering pharmacokinetic modifications with aging, which factors should be taken into consideration when evaluating Mrs. D's medication?

Pharmacokinetic changes should be considered when evaluating Mrs. D's medications. With aging, a decrease in renal function is reported. Mrs. D's creatinine clearance calculated using the Cockcroft and Gault formula is 30 mL/min. Medications that are renally excreted should be adjusted. Metformin in this case is contraindicated with a creatinine clearance of less than 30 ml/min. Metabolites of glyburide are also renally excreted and not indicated with a CrCl of less than 50 ml/min due to their accumulation and increased risk of hypoglycemia. Age-related changes with absorption, distribution, metabolism and elimination of medications with normal aging and in the frail elderly are described in the following table.

Age-related changes in pharmacokinetics with normal aging and in the frail elderly

	Age-related changes	Normal Aging	Frail elderly
Absorption	No changes	No clinical impact	⇓
Distribution	Body Fat	⇑ volume of distribution for liposoluble drugs. Adjust dosage for fat soluble drugs such as antipsychotics, antidepressants, benzodiazepines	⇑⇑
Distribution	Total water	⇓ Volume of distribution for water-soluble drugs. Adjust dosage for water-soluble drugs such as diuretics, digoxin, oral hypoglycemic	⇓⇓
	Albumin	⇓ Free fraction for drugs that are more than 90% bound to albumin such as phenytoin, valproic acid, warfarin	⇓⇓
Metabolism	Hepatic blood flow	⇓ First-pass extraction by the liver for drugs such as verapamil, propranolol.	⇓⇓
	Esterase enzymes	⇓ Metabolism of drugs metabolized by esterase enzymes. For ex: decreased metabolism of prodrug-enalapril to enalaprilat	⇓⇓
	Phase I metabolism	⇓ Metabolism of drugs metabolized by oxidation reaction	⇓⇓
	Phase II metabolism	No changes with normal aging	⇓ Changes in glucoronidation of acetaminophen and clearance of metoclopramide

Elimination	Glomerular filtration rate	⇓ Elimination of drugs renally excreted	⇓⇓
	Tubular secretion	⇓ Elimination of drugs excreted by tubular secretion such as cimetidine, trimethroprim	⇓⇓
	Serum creatinine	No changes with normal aging	⇓⇓ For low weight patient with decreased muscle mass, decrease in serum creatinine level
	Creatinine clearance	⇓ with normal aging	⇓

What are the therapeutic objectives for her diabetes and hypertension?

Considering her life expectancy and level of autonomy, therapeutic objectives for Hb A1c of < 8,5% and glucose level between 5 and 10 mmol/L would be appropriate for this patient to avoid hypoglycemia (cause of falls). Metformin and glyburide can be discontinued with close monitoring of blood glucose. Her daughter can be involved in documenting blood glucose for the next few weeks. If needed, another antidiabetic agent such as an inhibitor of the dipeptidyl peptidase-4 (DPP-4) can be prescribed.

For her hypertension, blood pressure goals should be less than 150/90 without orthostatic hypotension. Evaluation of orthostatic hypotension should therefore be done. If Mrs D has peripheral edema due to her amlodipine and was prescribed furosemide for this problem (medication cascade), these drugs should be discontinued. An angio-tensin-converting-enzyme inhibitor should be considered.

Why should drugs with anticholinergic properties be avoided in the elderly? Studies have shown that medications with anticholinergic properties have been associated with falls, and a decline in functional and cognitive capacity. A withdrawal plan should be implemented when stopping these medications. As discussed, Mrs D is taking Tylenol PM which has acet-aminophen and diphenhydramine as active ingredients. This should be stopped and discussion of the treatment of her "insomnia" initiated.

As per Beers Criteria for PIM, the following table illus-trates a list of medications with strong anticholinergic drugs that should be avoided in the elderly. The following table illustrates the most common anticholinergic drugs used in clinical practice.

Common drugs with anticholinergic properties as listed in AGS Updated Beers Criteria 2015

Antiemetic	Dimenhydrinate, promethazine
Antihistamines	Chlorpheniramine, cyproheptadine, diphenhydramine, hydroxyzine, meclizine
Antidepressants	Amitriptyline, desipramine, doxepin (>6 mg), nortriptyline, paroxetine
Antimuscarinics	Darifenacin, fesoterodine, oxytubynin, solifenacin, tolterodine, trospium
Antiparkinsonian	Benztropine, trihexyphenidyl

Antipsychotics	Cloxapine, loxapine, olanzapine
Antispasmodics	Atropine (excludes opthalmic), clidinium-chlordiazepoxide, dicyclomine, scopolamine
Skeletal muscle relaxants	Cyclobenzaprine, Methocarbamol, orphenadrine

Which drugs can be discontinued in Mrs D's case?

When the decision is made to implement a drug deprescribing plan, thus discontinuing medications, a plan should be put in place for monitoring and follow-up. This is an on-going re-evaluation. The following table illustrates the problems, drugs, therapeutic objectives and other considerations to evaluate if needed.

- For example, are the treatment goals achieved.
- Can a non pharmacological approach be implemented.
- Determine if you need to taper a medication.
- Supervision of drug discontinuation should be made by one physician. Collaboration can be made with community pharmacist for example to taper a benzodiazepine.

Match problems, drugs and therapeutic objectives

Problems	Current Drugs	Therapeutic objectives	Others
Falls	Tylenol PM	Pain control with acetaminophen alone	Gait evaluation and rehabilitation

Diabetes	Metformin 850 mg po bid Glyburide 5 mg po bid	HbA1c<8,5% Glucose between 5 and 10 mmol/L	
Hypertension	Amlodipine 5 mg daily Furosemide 40 mg daily	SBP < 150 without orthostatic hypotension	Moderate salt intake
Hypothyroidism	Levothyroxine 88 mcg po daily	TSH 0.4 and 4.4	Verify compliance
? GI	Pantoprazole 40 mg po daily	Clarify indication	Discontinue. Suggest looking at www. Deprescribing.org
? Cholesterol	Atorvastatin 40 mg po daily	Discontinue	
Depression	Citalopram 20 mg po daily	No clear indication	Geriatric Depression Scale
Insomnia	Lorazepam 1 mg po at bedtime	Better sleep	Sleep hygiene
Constipation	Docusate sodium 100 mg po bid	Regular bowel movement as per patient	Docusate sodium not effective long term. Change for Lax-a-day 17 g po daily

Conclusion

Evaluating medications in the elderly should be done on a regular basis, in order to modify risk factors to avoid geriatric syndromes such as falls, delirium etc. When prescribing a new medication to an elderly patient, the patient's expectations and preferences, and the objective of treatment according to life expectancy should be included in the discussion.

"It takes one minute to prescribe a medication but years to discontinue it."

Louise Mallet, February 2018.

Suggested reading

1. American Geriatrics Society 2015 Beers Criteria Update Expert Panel (2015) American Geriatrics Society 2015 updated Beers Criteria for potentially inappropriate medication use in older adults. J Am Geriatr Soc 63: 2227-2246

2. Bowles S. Polypharmacy. In: Huang A, Mallet L. ed. Medication-Related Falls in Older People: Causative Factors and Management Strategies. Springer Nature, Switzerland, 2016, p. 41-54.

3. Holmes, H. M. et al. Life expectancies predictions for women and men on the basis of US life tables. Arch Intern Med 2006; 166: 605-609

4. Reeve E, Shakib S, Hendrix I et al. Review of deprescribing processes and development of an evidence-based, patient-centred deprescribing process. Br J Clin Pharmcol 2014; 78: 738-747.

5. Scott IA, Hilmer SN, Reeve E et al. Reducing inappropriate polypharmacy. The process of deprescribing. JAMA Intern Med. 2015; 175: 827-834.

6. Holmes, H. M. et al. Life expectancies predictions for women and men on the basis of US life tables. Arch Intern Med 2006;166: 605-609

7. Mallet L. Pharmacology of Drugs in Aging. In: Huang A, Mallet L. ed. Medication-Related Falls in Older People: Causative Factors and Management Strategies. Springer Nature, Switzerland, 2016, p. 55-66.

8. Rochon P, Gurwitz JH. The prescribing cascade revisited. Lancet 2016; 389: 1778-1780.

ELDER ABUSE

Mark J. Yaffe, MDCM, MClSc, CCFP, FCFP
Professor, Department of Family Medicine
McGill University and St. Mary's Hospital Center

Clinical Vignette

Mrs. L is an eighty-eight year old widow with stable ischemic heart disease and diet-controlled Type 2 diabetes mellitus. She has shown gradual deterioration in short term memory and in judgment. She downplays deficits suggested by her MMSE score of 24, and is angry at her family doctor for notifying the license bureau about concerns about her ability to drive safely. Mrs. L. lives alone, with the exception of a housekeeper who comes to her apartment three half days per week to prepare some meals, do laundry, and to assist with bathing / hygiene. Mrs. L. downplays the need for the latter. The housekeeper had tried a number of times to attend to these issues, but in response to Mrs L.'s lack of cooperation the housekeeper became physically rough with the bathing. As well she has gradually ignored skin sores on the upper legs and buttocks.

Social contact with friends decreased over the preceding few years, aggravated by hearing loss. Following audiology testing Mrs. L. was advised that she would benefit from a particular hearing aid that would be easily useable, despite severe osteoarthritis in her hands. Mrs. L. stated that she could not afford the co-payment cost of the apparatus. The housekeeper frequently yells at her that she is too tight with her money, but Mrs. L. gives into frequent pleas from the housekeeper for extra money to help with troubled members of her family.

The family doctor has suggested a home visit by a community nurse or social worker, but this has been turned down by Mrs. L. She does, however, reluctantly give the physician permission to telephone her only child, a daughter who lives 2000 miles away. The latter is hard to reach and voice messages that are left are not returned. When contact is eventually made, the daughter indicates that she talks to her mother about once every three to four weeks, and that, while her mother might be a little eccentric, she was a "normal 88 year old who requires no new interventions. " The family physician learns that the daughter has power of attorney for mother's affairs, that she hasn't made much attempt to keep track of her mother's finances, and that she was unaware of money regularly being given to the homemaker independent of her usual pay.

What is elder abuse?

Elder abuse encompasses mistreatment and neglect of an older adult (in some communities the use of the word "elder" would be inappropriate as it might be a designation for a community leader of any age). Elder abuse represents single or multiple acts of commission or omission inflicted on an older adult (commonly viewed as aged 60 or 65, or older) within a relationship where there is an expectation of trust. (1) While mistreatment may occur as a result of ignorance, it is usually considered non-accidental or intentional, though intent to harm may in some cases be difficult to substantiate.

Elder abuse is important to detect and respond to not only to address the overt and sometimes covert sequelae of the mistreatment, but also to prolong the lives of the victims: Seniors who have been abused have a significantly higher mortality rate (independent of the abuse) when compared to seniors who have not been abused. (2)

Health care professionals may encounter older adults with signs and / or symptoms of abuse in varied settings: during home visits, in office settings, in emergency rooms, on acute care hospital wards, and in long term care institutions. Within the latter a distinction is encouraged between acts that are uniquely aimed at an individual (elder abuse) and those that may be due to institutional or systemic failure. Both are important to address, but solutions may rest at different levels of care.

As described below elder abuse is commonly divided into four categories: physical, psychological / verbal, financial / material, and neglect (3) :

Physical abuse
Acts associated with physical abuse include:

- Individuals who are hit, slapped, kicked, tied, shaken, choked, grabbed, pushed , shoved, punched, slammed against a wall, pinched, scratched, bit, burned, scalded
- Twisted limbs
- Rough transfers
- Unexplained or poorly explained falls and injuries
- Multiple visits to emergency departments
- Use of a weapon
- Improper use of physical or chemical restraint
- Sexual Abuse: Unwanted sexual contact, touching, or rubbing; Masturbation that is forced, tricked, coerced, manipulated; use of physical threats (hitting, holding down, use of weapon) to give or receive oral, genital, or anal sex

Manifestations of physical abuse: Unexplained or unusual
- Bruises (especially those that are finger or knuckle shaped)
- Need for new dental work
- Lacerations, abrasions, scars
- Sprains, fractures, multiple trauma
- Genital inflammation, pain, tenderness
- Signs of anxiety, depression, withdrawal, low eye contact

Psychological/verbal abuse

Acts associated with psychological abuse include
- Lying
- Humiliating or infantilizing
- Demeaning talk or jokes
- Coercion
- Inappropriate shouting / yelling
- Controlling verbal or physical contact with family or friends
- Threatening to hit or throw something
- Disrespect for privacy
- Insulting, swearing, name calling, putting down
- Threats with weapons, deprivation, punishment, guardianship, abandonment, institutionalization
- Sexual: Verbal threats to give or receive oral, genital, or anal sex; individuals forced to view or

participate in pornographic or sexually explicit pictures or videos; offensive sexual talk

Manifestations of psychological abuse: Unexplained or unusual
- Apprehensiveness
- Physical avoidance
- Reduced eye contact or continual eye darting
- Quietness, passivity, withdrawal
- Depression, anger
- Weight loss
- Missed appointments
- Caregivers who try to answer in place of the senior

Financial or material abuse
Acts associated with financial / material abuse include
- Disrespect for property, including taking, misuse, concealment of resources, property, or assets, with or without coercion, enticement, intimidation, or deception
- Misappropriation of funds, bank accounts, or credit/ debit cards against the will of a senior or without his/her knowledge
- Forced to give power of attorney,
- Forged signature
- Use of power attorney or employment of service people by others for personal gain

Manifestations of financial / material abuse: Unexplained or unusual

- Anxiety, apprehensiveness, avoidance
- Social withdrawal
- Depression, tearfulness, weight loss
- Clothes not appropriate to the weather
- Under-medicated

Neglect

Acts associated with neglect include

- Inappropriately left alone or unsupervised
- Withholding of necessary aides: walker, wheel-chair, glasses, hearing aid, telephone
- Living environment too hot or too cold
- Clothing inappropriate to weather
- Unsanitary living conditions, bed linens or incontinence products not changed
- Medications not or irregularly supervised
- Inappropriate or poor food supplied
- Delays in seeking treatment
- Inconsistent treatment
- Frequent change of physicians

Manifestations of neglect:

- Poor mobility
- Cachexia
- Decubitus ulcers, pressure sores, bed sores

- Poor hygiene, body odor
- Frequent infections
- Unexplained medical problems
- Fearfulness, anxiety, depression

Systemic or Institutional Failure

Acts associated with institutional or systemic failure include

- Inadequate custodial care or supervision
- Low or unpredictable nursing/nursing aide care
- Delays in response time to seniors' calls for help
- Inadequate nutrition
- Overcrowded or unsanitary living conditions
- Poor staff communication skills
- Limited staff language competency
- Recurrent inappropriate staff- resident interactions
- Misuse of physical or chemical restraints

Detection of elder abuse

Risk Factors

Since physicians of varied backgrounds and experience may be the first or enduring point of contact for an abused senior, a knowledge of elder abuse is promoted despite sometimes vague signs and symptoms. Guidelines are neither for or against whether physicians should routinely screen for elder abuse. Research into risk factors has generated some of this uncertainty because of a lack of clarity about their impact. Nonetheless it is useful to be aware of such factors and the roles they may play in relation to elder abuse when considered from the perspectives of caregivers (CG) and care receivers (CR) (4):

Weak association	Moderate association	Strong association
Social isolation (CR)	Females (CR)	Poor physical health (CR)
Dementia (CR)	Blacks (CR)	Childhood violence (CG)
Mental illness (CG)	Passive/dependent (CR)	Stress (CG)
Hostility (CG)	CG dependent on CR	CR dependent on CG
Drugs / alcohol (CG)	CG related to CR	Institutional care (CG)

Detection instruments

There are a small number of validated detection tools for use by clinicians. (5) The Elder Abuse Suspicion Index (EASI) © is a practical one because its six questions take only 2-5 minutes to complete. (6) The self-administered version, the EASI-sa, is comprised of 5 questions and is completed in a similar brief time frame. (7) These tools use words understandable by, and acceptable to, older adults (7), and is available in ten languages. (8) A nine question tool derived from the EASI has been specifically designed for use in the long term care setting (EASI-ltc), and is pending formal testing. (9) Copies of the Elder Abuse Suspicion Index tools and practical aspects of their application are found on a website devoted to it: http://www.mcgill.ca/familymed/research/projects/elder

Outcome of suspected abuse

Since a positive response on the EASI can be a false positive arising from cognitive impairment (delirium, dementia), a MMSE (or equivalent tool) should be performed as part of a mental capacity assessment, the EASI being validated for cognition scores of ≥ 24 on the MMSE. If the senior is found by this process to be inapt, then a declaration of such should be made according to the reporting protocol of the jurisdiction in which one is practicing.

Does identification of elder abuse by a cognitively intact senior legally bind a physician to report the mistreatment? It depends on the geographical jurisdiction in which one is practicing. Some do not impose mandatory reporting; some require it for abuse that occurs within a public institution that cares for seniors; and others require reporting irrespective of where the abuse has occurred. A dilemma for practitioners is that some cognitively intact victims do not want the abuse disclosed. There may be reluctance to see the abuser punished; they may be embarrassed, humiliated, or shamed that a family member was abusive; they may fear retaliation from the abuser; or they may realistically worry that removing the abuser may leave their global living situations worse than it was with the abuse.

Such situations are legally and ethically challenging. It would therefore be advisable for clinicians to seek the advice and collaboration of regionally designated resources for elder abuse: Adult Protective Services, social services, or police officers. What can health professionals expect from these experts? Where feasible, social workers will do a complete evaluation of the psychosocial needs of the older person and the caregiver. If indicated, along with a doctor's help, they will begin procedures to have the person declared under a protective regime (public, private curatorship, or homologation of a mandate). They will access homecare services, respite programs, caregiver support groups and placement, if necessary. If the senior is competent, they will respect the right of self- determination, but support the person to have a life without abuse. If indicated, they will involve the police or get a Human Right's Commission (or equivalent) involved.

Clinical vignette continued

The case history described self-neglect; self-neglect, however, does not appear in the cited descriptors of elder abuse. It is considered a different problem, with causes and possible solutions that require a unique approach. The vignette does however suggest neglect on the part of the homemaker and the out-of-town daughter. It does provide evidence of verbal as well as physical abuse by the homemaker. Both daughter and homemaker appear to be abusing the trust mother had in them as far as her finances were concerned.

In the vignette the family physician has not directly used a detection tool to gather data; however he has taken advantage of his knowledge of the content of the EASI to ask Mrs. L. and her daughter relevant questions. As a result he feels more urgency in the situation and in a need to get help for Mrs. L. He reminds her that over his 22 years of care for her that he had tried to respect her best interests. Responding positively to this reminder she agrees to have a visit from a social worker, but reserves the right to keep open whatever options may be available to her.

References

1. World Health Organization. *The Toronto declaration on the global prevention of elder abuse.* Geneva, Switzerland: World Health Organization; 2002.
2. Lachs MS, Williams CS, O'Brien S, Pillemer KA, Chartlson ME. *The mortality of elder mistreatment.* JAMA 1998; 280 (5)428-32.
3. Yaffe MJ, Tazkarji B. *Understanding elder abuse in family practice.* Canadian Family Physician 2012; 58: 1336-40.
4. Yaffe MJ. *Elder Abuse.* Chapter in Calhoun K, Eibling DE, Wax MK, Kost K. Geriatric Otolaryngology. Taylor and Francis, New York, 2006. P 639.
5. McMullen T, Schwartz K, Yaffe M, Beach S. *Elder Abuse and Its Prevention: Screening and detection,* IOM (Institute of Medicine) and NRC

(National Research Council: Elder Abuse and Its Prevention: Workshop Summary, pp: 88-93, The National Academies Press Washington, DC, April 2014.

6. Yaffe MJ, Wolfson C, Weiss D, Lithwick M. *Development and validation of a tool to assist physicians' identification of elder abuse: The Elder Abuse Suspicion Index (EASI ©)*. Journal of Elder Abuse and Neglect, 2008; 20 (3): 276-300.

7. Yaffe MJ, Weiss D, Lithwick M. *Seniors' Self-Administration of the Elder Abuse Suspicion Index (EASI): A Feasibility Study. Journal of Elder Abuse and Neglect* 2012; 24 (2) 277-292.

8. http://www.mcgill.ca/familymed/research/projects/elder

9. Ballard SA, Yaffe MJ, August L, Cetin-Sahin D, Wilchesky M. Adapting the Elder Abuse Suspicion Index © for use in long-term care: A mixd methods approach. Journal of Applied Gerontology. In press, June 2017.

MANAGEMENT OF OLDER PATIENTS IN THE EMERGENCY DEPARTMENT: THIS MAN IS OLD, BUT IS IT AN EMERGENCY?

Cyrille Launay, MD, PhD, Department of medicine, division of geriatrics, University Hospital of Lausanne, Switzerland

Clinical vignette

An 88 year old man is brought to the emergency department (ED) by his daughter because he can no longer perform his basic activities of daily living (bathing, dressing, transferring). She also reports that her father was having difficulty preparing his meals and has lost weight. The patient cannot provide details and does not understand why he is at hospital. He has no complaints and states that even if he is "a little bit tired", he wants to go back home. He is coherent but he is not able to say the month or the year. He has a mild cough but has no fever. The chest examination reveals wheezing but no audible crackles. Blood tests available disclose leukocytes $7x10^9$/L, CRP 15mg/L, creatinine 67 umol/L. The physician diagnoses acute bronchitis, proposes discharge home and treatment with an opioid cough suppressant.

Why are older patients in the Emergency Department at risk of misdiagnosis?

The health status of older patients (i.e; 75 years and older) is highly heterogeneous and is related to the various and cumulative effects of aging, life habits and chronic diseases that are highly prevalent in this age group. Thus, older patients are generally sicker than younger ones and 80% of those aged 75 years and older present with at least 2 chronic diseases that increase the risk of developing acute diseases. Indeed, older patients often experience complex interactions between acute and chronic diseases but also geriatric syndromes (e.g., cognitive impairment) that may induce atypical clinical presentations such as functional decline or increasing disabilities. Thus, they may be admitted to ED with non-specific complaints (feeling "tired" or "weak") that arise due to cognitive impairment and communications problems, functional decline and co-morbidities. Geriatric syndromes may not be recognized (misdiagnosed) and not managed (mistreated).

Therefore, 25% of older patients leave ED with no definite diagnosis whereas most of them suffer from an acute disease. Underdiagnosis and underestimation of patients with atypical clinical presentations may lead to adverse outcomes such as higher risk of hospitalization and in-hospital mortality.

How to deal with older patients in the Emergency Department

The adapted care plan of older patients is based on a multidimensional, interdisciplinary diagnostic process to determine the medical, psychological and functional capabilities called the comprehensive geriatric assessment (CGA). CGA is the most validated intervention dedicated to elderly patients and aims at assessing and addressing their needs.

Benefits of CGA have been confirmed through several meta-analysis, which have reported a reduction of admissions and readmissions to hospital, more discharges to home, increased lifetime spent at home, prevention of functional decline and decrease in mortality and in healthcare expenditures.

Despite its benefits, a systematic CGA for every older ED inpatient in daily practice remains impossible to implement because it is a complex and time-consuming process. Furthermore, it requires a multidisciplinary geriatric team that cannot alone support the care of all frail older ED patients due to limited availability.

The usual Emergency Department's mission is to quickly prioritize patients whose life is in danger; therefore, their triage often fails to detect the complex reasons that lead to the ED visits of older patients.

Thus, a two-step approach seems the best strategy to provide the appropriate care to the right patient at the right time, in order to identify those who are in greatest need of a geriatric intervention.

To implement such an approach, a screening tool is required to identify frail patients or patients at risk of adverse outcomes during hospitalization.

Useful tools to identify vulnerable patients in ED

Several tools have been developed to identify early frail patients or patients at risk of a prolonged hospital stay, 30-day readmission or mortality. There is currently no consensus on a screening tool for use in ED. The ideal tool would need to be multidimensional. Thus, most of the screening tools in use assess physical function, cognition, malnutrition and disabilities that are the main geriatric conditions.

To date, there is a consensus for the need for a screening tool in ED, but this tool needs to be adapted to the specific conditions of the medical practice in ED. This tool needs to be multidimensional, capable of being quickly performed and easy to use without specific geriatric training. Among those tools, Identification of Senior At Risk (ISAR), Emergency Room Evaluation and Recommendations (ER2) or Prisma

7 are meant to guide the appropriate levels of treatment to provide to older patients. According to their risk stratification, patients considered frail or at risk of prolonged length of hospital stay may require a geriatric intervention (i.e; to be hospitalized in a geriatric unit, or the intervention of a mobile geriatric team).

Key components of a comprehensive geriatric assessment	
Medical assessment	Problem list Comorbidities Medications Nutritional assessment Gait and balance assessment
Functional assessment	Activities of daily living Instrumental activities of daily living
Psychological assessment	Cognition Assessment of mood
Social Assessment	Family support Home help services
environmental assessment	Financial

If no screening tool is available, an assessment based on the components of the CGA may be performed.

CGA allows a coordinated and integrated plan of treatment, and thus may prevent complicated medical pathways characterized, for instance, by prolonged length of hospital stay. This intervention can be performed in different ways depending on the medical resources and organization of the structure. Most of the time, CGA is delivered on a geriatric ward, or by a mobile geriatric team.

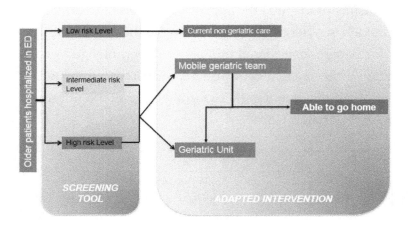

In EDs, mobile geriatric assessment provides an intervention with several objectives. The first one is to diagnose unrecognized geriatric syndromes such as delirium, frailty and gait impairment. Secondly, the mobile geriatric team may provide guidance on the level of care and recommendations on immediate care, prevention of functional decline or prevention of delirium. Finally, mobile geriatric teams may propose and coordinate a care plan that includes a discharge home or suggest the type of inpatient medical unit that may provide the most adapted care (e.g., a geriatric unit, an internal medicine unit) or institutionalization.

Continuation of the vignette

A mobile geriatric team is asked to assess the patient in order to help with the medical management and to coordinate the discharge.

Their geriatric assessment uncovers several geriatric syndromes. First, cognitive impairment is detected, using the Mini Mental State Examination (MMSE). Secondly, they gather information that the patient fell many times and always refused a walking aid. Finally, malnutrition is diagnosed considering a weight loss of 7kg in the last 6 months and a lower than expected weight of 61kg. The mobile geriatric team provided a plan for immediate care and proposed to transfer the patient to an acute geriatric unit.

How to deliver a geriatric assessment in ED?

Several areas must be considered to assess older patients. These areas have been grouped under the acronym of 5Ms as proposed by the American and Canadian Geriatrics Societies. These 5 Ms stand for:

- **Mind: refers to cognitive impairment and/or delirium and depression:** Delirium is highly prevalent in EDs (up to a quarter of patients) and should not remain unrecognized considering related morbidity and adverse outcomes. The confusion assessment method (CAM) is a simple tool with high predictive performance that may be used to identify delirium. Patients with cognitive impairment are vulnerable and must be managed carefully because of the risk of delirium. Besides, assessing their cognitive status is mandatory to enable a safe return home from ED. For interventions to reduce or manage delirium, please refer to the chapter on delirium.

- **Mobility: refers to gait impairment and falls:** Half of those aged 80 years and over fall at least once a year. Thus the history of falls is a predictor of future falls and is also associated with greater disabilities and injuries. The intervention may assess the risk of falls and identify their risk factors, in order to implement multidisciplinary interventions to address them. For details on the management of mobility and falls in older adults, please refer to the dedicated chapter.

- **Multi-complexity: refers to the burden of chronic diseases and bio-psycho-social situations including functional status:** Functional decline and disabilities are relatively common reasons for visits to EDs by older patients and may be the clinical presentation of an underlying disease. That is why such non-specific complaints must trigger an exhaustive assessment of acute and chronic diseases and geriatric syndromes.

- **Medication: refers to optimization of prescriptions and adverse drug events.** Taking 5 different medications or more per day usually defines polypharmacy. Adverse drug effects increase with aging and number of drugs and may be a reason for ED visits in up to 14% of older persons. Furthermore, the number of drugs taken per day is associated with comorbidity burden and diseases' severity. For more information on polypharmacy, please refer to the appropriate chapter.

- **Matters most: refers to each individual's own meaningful health outcome goals and care preferences.** These important aspects can be discussed with the caregiver when the patient is unable to contribute. Emphasis should be placed on patient-centered care.

Resolution of the clinical vignette

Many geriatric syndromes may be evoked from the beginning of this vignette. The reason for admission is non-specific and the clinical presentation is mainly functional. Such a visit could be considered inappropriate in ED whose aim is intended to treat acute diseases. However, nearly 60% of patients presenting with non-specific complaints to ED suffer from serious medical conditions. Acute functional decline may lead to disabilities. It is mandatory to provide specific interventions that improve the diagnostic process to manage patients adequately and prevent further decline. The main clinical elements suggest acute bronchitis without severity criteria. However an acute disease may expose a vulnerable patient with reduced physiological reserves to dependency.

The patient is described as not able to say the month or the year, suggestive of cognitive impairment. Indeed, temporal disorientation is related to acute and chronic cognitive impairment. Thus this item may help to identify delirium and/or dementia. Consequently, opioid treatment must be used with caution to avoid delirium and is not indicated to treat cough. A brief geriatric assessment that examines cognition is mandatory in this case. Confirmation of a diagnosis of dementia can be completed at a later stage along with a decision on treatment.

Finally, this clinical vignette shows the necessity to go beyond the assessment of acute diseases in ED and to consider geriatric syndromes and chronic diseases. A care plan to prevent functional decline, disabilities and delirium must be elaborated from ED to avoid inappropriate discharge home with its deleterious consequences.

References

Preston L et al. Southampton (UK): NIHR Journals Library; 2018

Ellis G, Whitehead MA, O'Neill D, Langhorne P, Robinson D. Comprehensive geriatric assessment for older adults admitted to hospital. Cochrane Database Syst Rev. 2011;doi: 10.1002/14651858.

Aminzadeh F, Dalziel WB. Older adults in the emergency department: a systematic review of patterns of use, adverse outcomes, and effectiveness of interventions. Ann Emerg Med. 2002;39:238-247.

Wachelder JJH, Stassen PM, Hubens LPAM et al. Elderly patients presenting with non -specific complaints: characteristics and outcomes. PlosOne.2017; 12(11): e0188954

Ellis G, Marshall T, Ritchie C. Comprehensive geriatric assessment in the emergency department. Clin Interv Aging. 2014; 9: 2033–2043.

Sternberg SA, Wershof Schwartz A, Karunananthan S, Bergman H, Mark Clarfield A. The identification of frailty: a systematic literature review.J Am Geriatr Soc. **2011 Nov;59(11):2129-38.**

AN OVERVIEW OF LATE-LIFE DEPRESSION

Artin Mahdanian, MD, MSc; Silvia Monti De Flores, MD, FRCPC, DFAPA
Department of Psychiatry, McGill University

Clinical vignette

Mr. D is a 73-year-old divorced man who was brought to the emergency room by his daughter for suicidal ideation and depression. He described a few months' history of continuous excessive worry about his future, panic attacks and loss of interest in life. He self-isolated and avoided seeing family and friends. He had gradually stopped all of the physical exercise activities (swimming, jogging and yoga) that he used to do, because he did not have the physical energy and mental joy. He had difficulty sleeping, decreased appetite and had lost about 10 pounds in the past few months. Recently, he had been feeling very guilty about how he had treated his ex-wife who died of suicide by hanging 20 years ago, 10 years after their divorce. He thought he deserved to die and started to think about ending his life. He denied any delusions or hallucinations. He did not have any anxiety or other psychiatric symptoms prior to this episode except for few months of "psychotherapy" with a psychologist 30 years ago after his divorce.

His symptoms started a few months ago when his company went bankrupt following a few months of struggling with a tax audit and numerous financial problems. Then, he decided to retire. He used to be a very successful and high-achieving accountant who ran the company with his brother for more than 40 years. He suffers from diabetes mellitus type II, gout and a frozen shoulder. His medication list includes Vitamin B12, Metformin-Sitagliptin 1000mg+50mg, Valsartan-HCTZ 160mg+25mg, and Allopurinol. The only important family history was chronic treatment-resistant depression in his mother.

What is depression?

Depression is a general term which is used for Major Depressive Disorder (MDD). Diagnosis is always a clinical one and it is based on meeting the diagnostic criteria for either DSM-5 or ICD-10. For the diagnosis of MDD based on DSM-5, there must be 5 symptoms; one of them should be either depressed mood or lack of interest (anhedonia) and 4 other symptoms out of psychomotor slowness, decreased/increased appetite, weight changes, sleep disturbances, suicidal ideation, decreased energy, decreased concentration, or feeling guilty. The symptoms must be persistent and present most of the time for a period of at least two weeks. Moreover, there should be a decline in baseline functioning of the patient.

Why is depression an important clinical problem in the elderly?

MDD is one of the most common causes of disability worldwide. It is a highly prevalent disorder characterized by episodes of persistent depressed mood or loss of interest/pleasure (affective symptoms) plus other vegetative and cognitive symptoms as described above.

Late-life depression (LLD), with an estimated prevalence of about 15%, is a common psychiatric disorder in people >65y. LLD is associated with increased morbidity and mortality. It is associated with increased healthcare cost. LLD has also been shown to be highly recurrent with research reports varying between 30% and 65% over 3 to 20 years follow-up. The consequences of untreated LLD include poor quality of life as well as worse outcome and exacerbation of other chronic illnesses, and most importantly, suicide.

Predictors of poorer outcome may include adverse childhood events, age of onset, limited education, and the number of previous recurrences and length of untreated episodes. Additionally, personality disorder diagnosis (avoidant, obsessive compulsive, and introvert personality traits) may predict a further episode, while somatoform disorders may predict time to recurrence. Due to the atypical presentation, the diagnosis of LLD is often missed by primary care physicians, which leads to under-treatment of the disease. However, a timely diagnosis can be life-saving and, when treated, it has a good prognosis; up to 70% of treated older patients achieve full remission.

What are the challenges in diagnosis of depression in the elderly?

In the geriatric population, depressive symptoms may be masked by unexplained physical complaints (e.g., fatigue, diffuse pain or back pain, headache, chest pain, etc.) and, subsequently, the classical DSM 5 criteria may sometimes seem to fail in terms of diagnosing depression. Furthermore, the conditions mentioned below can exist concomitantly.

Therefore, the differential diagnosis of LLD in the elderly is broad including, but not limited to, Central Nervous System disorders (dementia, Parkinson disease, and neoplastic lesions), other psychiatric disorders (dysthymia, bipolar, and anxiety disorders), endocrine disorders (hypo-hyperthyroidism, and hyperparathyroidism), medication side effects (e.g., β-blockers, centrally active antihypertensive medications, steroids, H2-blockers, sedatives, certain chemotherapy agents), vitamin deficiency (vitamin B12, vitamin D, and folic acid), life circumstances (e.g., grief, bereavement, financial or autonomy losses), substance use, infectious and inflammatory diseases (e.g., HIV encephalopathy, systemic lupus erythematosus) and sleep disorders (in particular, obstructive sleep apnea).

A complete physical examination, cognitive screening, laboratory tests and/or imaging are the first steps in ruling out these differential diagnoses and in assessing for common comorbidities in the elderly. A physician who has good understanding of the patient's personality can identify nonverbal cues and changes in behavior indicating mood problems. In addition, information from family members and caregivers on the patient's mood and behavior is vital for assessing the older person with depression.

What are the risk factors for depression?

As in all other aspects of depression, the risk factors for LLD are also better described in a biopsychosocial model. The main biological risk factors are old age and female sex. In addition, genetic vulnerability also plays an important role, making people with family history of mood disorders more susceptible to LLD than others. Patients with poor physical health (e.g. multiple comorbidities, sleeping disorders, etc.) and more medication use may also be predisposed to LLD. The notion of frailty affects several domains of functioning, leading to a deterioration in the resilience and capacity for dealing with stressors. Frailty can be defined by the Fried criteria: weight loss, decreased handgrip strength, slowness, exhaustion, and low physical activity. Poor nutritional status is also associated with frailty and LLD; therefore, nutritional supplements (vitamins D, B12, folate and protein) could benefit the depressed frail patient. Neurodegenerative disease (e.g., Parkinson or Alzheimer) and mild cognitive impairment (MCI) are also considered possible risk factors for LLD. We know that LLD and dementia frequently co-occur, and depression can be the first sign of dementia. The vascular hypothesis holds that cerebrovascular disease may cause or predispose to LLD and can be explained by reduced cerebral perfusion, altered brain connectivity, and chronic low-grade inflammation.

Psychological factors such as loss of purpose in life or human relationships seem to be associated with LLD. Moreover, lower level of education, being a widower or single, loneliness, lack of social supports, stressful life events and poverty are all valid risk factors for LLD. Decrease or loss of functional status, visual or hearing impairment, poor lifestyle habits, smoking and alcohol use also increase the risk of developing LLD. In addition, the use of sleep medication such as benzodiazepines and sleep disturbance in general are also correlated with increased risk of LLD.

Useful tools for the diagnosis of depression?

Use of validated scales/tools in screening, diagnosis, and follow-up response to therapy in depression is an important part of providing appropriate care. They can improve diagnostic accuracy, save time, provide more consistent patient care, and monitor a patient's complex emotional and behavioral responses to therapy. Two quick questions from Primary Care Evaluation of Mental Disorders can provide us with a highly sensitive (94%) but not very specific (35%) screening test for depression: 1. Have you been bothered by little interest or pleasure in doing things? 2. Have you been feeling down, depressed, or hopeless in the last month?

If a patient responds positively to either of these two questions, we can screen with the other symptom criteria. Other useful Self- or physician-rated screening tools are also available. The Hamilton Depression Rating Scale (HAM-D), the oldest, most widely used and validated instrument, has numerous versions, both clinician-rated and self-reported, as well as a computer administered version. Many clinicians prefer to use a patient rated scale such as the Beck Depression Inventory (BDI). The BDI has high sensitivity and specificity and is valid and reliable in assessing the severity of depressive symptoms. The Geriatric Depression Scale (GDS) is also a self-report measure designed to minimize the impact of somatic symptoms associated with aging and illness. It has good sensitivity and positive predictive values for diagnosis of major depression. The PHQ-9 also offers a severity score for symptoms, and can also be used to follow outcome. If a clinician is concerned about cognitive impairment, the Mini Mental State Exam (MMSE) and/or Montreal Cognitive Assessment (MoCA) are useful additions.

How is the diagnosis of depression conveyed to the patient?

There is no gold standard for discussing depression diagnosis with elderly patients. It is dependent on the physician's method since research on the topic is lacking. It is helpful to engage the patient with the use of the bio-psychosocial model: inform the patient that the illness is an interaction between physiological (e.g. neurotransmitters hypothesis like serotonin), psychological, and social factors. Creating a good therapeutic alliance and trust is pivotal for a good outcome.

What are the treatment options for depression?

The very first step in the treatment of depression is to treat the modifiable risk factors including nutritional deficiencies (vitamin B12, D, and folic acid), cardiovascular diseases, and any endocrine and electrolyte abnormalities. Risk factors can also be improved by lifestyle changes, physical exercise, healthy diet, sufficient sleep, smoking cessation, discontinuation of alcohol intake as well as optimal treatment for hypertension, hypercholesterolemia, hyperglycemia, and any other comorbid medical condition.

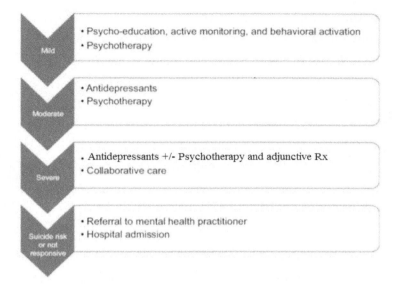

Figure 1. Stepped care approach to late-life depression, based on the severity of depression and patient preference

The treatment options of MDD are based on the bio-psychosocial model and the administered choice is according to the severity of the illness and patient preference (figure 1). The severity of the illness is defined based on rating scales, functional impairment and clinical impression. Biological treatments include pharmacotherapy with antidepressants, second generation antipsychotics, neuro-modulation approaches like Repetitive Transcranial Magnetic Stimulation (rTMS), electroconvulsive therapy (ECT), light therapy and supplements (Omega 3, Vit B12). Psychotherapeutic approaches with significant evidence for efficacy include: Supportive Psychotherapy, Cognitive Behavioural Therapy (CBT), Interpersonal Therapy (IPT), Mindfulness-Based Cognitive Therapy (MBCT), Life Review Therapy, Problem-solving Therapy (PST), Bibliotherapy (mostly based on CBT models), Dynamic Therapy, and Existential Therapy. Finally, Social interventions play an important role in treatment of depression in the elderly since losses, loneliness, social isolation, and a limited support network are very common in this population.

Psycho-education: The physician's role is to help patient understand depression, to explain therapeutic options, discuss the bio-psychosocial model of etiology and treatment, to recognize warning signs, and to inform and support the family. Moreover, it is important to try to provide a structure in the patient's life and activate the patient through structured and fun activities.

Behavioral activation: Structured physical activity is recommended for older people with mild or moderate depression who are physically capable.

Psychotherapy: Psychotherapies are the most important type of non-pharmacological treatment and are not inferior to pharmacological treatments in mild to moderate depression. Evidence-based psychotherapeutic treatments of depression in older adults include CBT, IPT, PST, and life review therapy.

Pharmacological treatment: Geriatric patients have different pharmacodynamics and pharmacokinetics due to age-related physiological changes. Therefore, despite the fact that treatment options and algorithms are the same as for other adults, the medications must be administered at lower doses and slowly titrated while actively monitoring the patient. Increased caution is necessary for drug interactions and polypharmacy. In addition, when choosing a psychotropic drug, keep track of the drug's safety profile since some adverse reactions like falls can lead to increased morbidity and mortality. Selective serotonin reuptake inhibitors (SSRIs), Serotonin–norepinephrine reuptake inhibitors (SNRIs), tricyclic antidepressants (TCAs), and atypical antidepressants are the main pharmacological treatments of choice. Existing evidence unanimously suggests that no one class of antidepressant drugs has been found to be more effective than another in the treatment of LLD. However, newer antidepressants are better tolerated and safer. When choosing an SSRI, slight preference goes to an SSRI with the least known drug interactions such as sertraline. TCAs are as effective as SSRIs for LLD, but are less often used because of side effects. TCAs with lesser anticholinergic side effects, such as nortriptyline, are more recommended. SNRIs are not only effective against depression but also effective in the treatment of peripheral neuropathic pain.

An atypical antidepressant that can be used as an alternative for SSRIs is mirtazapine. The sedative side effects of mirtazapine are used as a treatment for insomnia. In addition, mirtazapine increases the appetite and can be used for the symptom of anorexia. Other atypical antidepressants which are commonly used are Bupropion, Vortioxetine and Trazodone.

How Do You Manage Inadequate Response to an Antidepressant?

If a patient has partial or no response to the initial treatment, clinicians should ensure the dose of the medication is optimized to the therapeutic level as much as tolerated (6-8 weeks). There is extensive evidence that shows many patients receive sub-therapeutic doses and/or inadequate duration of treatment.

Evidence shows that switching non-responders to another antidepressant in the same class or another class results in good response and remission rates. However, patients with partial response to the initial antidepressant might benefit from increasing the dose and then the addition of a second medication; i.e. adjunctive treatment which means either combination (adding a second antidepressant to the first) or augmentation (adding another medication that is not an antidepressant, e.g., second generation antipsychotics, mood stabilizers like lithium, triiodothyronine).

Resolution of the clinical vignette

Having confirmed the diagnosis of MDD by a comprehensive history and physical exam, a full blood work up was done that turned out to be negative for other causes or comorbid conditions with MDD as indicated above. Mr. D was then started on Venlafaxine XR 37.5mg daily. In addition to providing him with psycho-education and support, it was suggested that he restart his physical exercise routine and socialize as much as possible. In the first follow-up visit after 1 week his response to medication and absence of side effects was assessed. His blood pressure and heart rate were monitored and found to to be normal. The dose of the medication was increased to 75mg daily. Mr. D returned in 2 weeks with some response to medication but still far from his baseline. The dose of the medication was slowly increased to 150mg daily. After about 6 weeks on the therapeutic dose of Venlafaxine, Mr. D still complained of some residual depressed mood, decreased energy and sleep disturbances despite some further improvement. At that point the treatment was augmented by adding Quetiapine 50mg at night and the dose very slowly increased to 100mg. When Mr. D was reassessed a few weeks later, he reported that he was completely back to his baseline in terms of mood and interest. He registered in the local community center for Yoga classes twice weekly, went swimming with his friends every other day, and travelled to visit his daughter for one week. He was advised to continue the treatment for 9-12 months as this was the first episode of depression and to taper down the treatment under supervision of a physician to avoid withdrawal symptoms and decrease the risk of relapse.

References

Physical exercise for late-life depression: Effects on symptom dimensions and time course. Murri MB, Ekkekakis P, Menchetti M, Neviani F, Trevisani F, Tedeschi S, Latessa PM, Nerozzi E, Ermini G, Zocchi D, Squatrito S, Toni G, Cabassi A, Neri M, Zanetidou S, Amore M. J Affect Disord. 2018 Apr 1;230:65-70. doi: 10.1016/j.jad.2018.01.004

Advances in Pharmacotherapy of Late-Life Depression. Beyer JL, Johnson KG. Curr Psychiatry Rep. 2018 Apr 7;20(5):34. doi: 10.1007/s11920-018-0899-6. Review.

Late-life depression: issues for the general practitioner. Van Damme A, Declercq T, Lemey L, Tandt H, Petrovic M. Int J Gen Med. 2018 Mar 29;11:113-120.

Treatment-resistant Late-life Depression: Challenges and Perspectives. Knöchel C, Alves G, Friedrichs B, Schneider B, Schmidt-Rechau A, Wenzler S, Schneider A, Prvulovic D, Carvalho AF, Oertel-Knöchel V. Curr Neuropharmacol. 2015;13(5):577-91.

Canadian Network for Mood and Anxiety Treatments (CANMAT) 2016 Clinical Guidelines for the Management of Adults with Major Depressive Disorder: Section 3. Pharmacological Treatments. Kennedy SH, Lam RW, McIntyre RS, Tourjman SV, Bhat V, Blier P, Hasnain M, Jollant F, Levitt AJ, MacQueen GM, McInerney SJ, McIntosh D, Milev RV, Müller DJ, Parikh SV, Pearson NL, Ravindran AV, Uher R; CANMAT Depression Work Group. Can J Psychiatry. 2016 Sep;61(9):540-60.

ASSESSMENT OF DECISION-MAKING CAPACITY

Catherine Ferrier, MD, Assistant Professor, Department of Family Medicine, Faculty of Medicine, McGill University

Vignette

Don is an 83-year-old retired engineer who presents with a one year history of cognitive symptoms. He forgets people's names and conversations he has had, and loses his keys. He lives with his wife; their two children live in the U.S. He remains independent for all basic and instrumental activities of daily living. He scores 29/30 on the MMSE and 27/30 on the MoCA. Some chronic ischemia is noted on brain CT. Laboratory tests are normal. A diagnosis of mild cognitive impairment is made.

He returns for follow-up 6 months later. His wife reports new spatial disorientation and difficulty understanding the use of electronic devices. He got lost once, so has stopped driving. The MMSE score is 22 and the MoCA 21. A diagnosis of mixed AD/vascular dementia is made and he is started on treatment with donepezil. You assess his capacity to assign a general power of attorney and a protection mandate.

A protection mandate in Quebec allows an individual to name someone or several people to take care of personal needs and property management upon incapacity. It is similar to an Advance Directive in the United States which is governed through different statutes in each state: see Chapter "How Do I Protect My Patient?" In other parts of Canada, documents analogous to a protection mandate may go by other names such as powers of attorney or representation agreement. It is important to consult with a qualified professional, usually an attorney, in the jurisdiction where the individual lives to ensure that documentation is correctly done.

It would appear that a protection mandate can be appointed by an individual in the event of future incapacity which is then determined by the appropriate health care provider. The protection mandate would become effective when homologated by the Court, specifically when a judgment is obtained regarding incapacity . In the United States, an Advance Directive can generally be put in place in order to avoid a Guardianship proceeding.

Don fully understands the concept and content of both documents. He signs them shortly after seeing you, naming his wife as a mandatary, the person appointed to act under the protection mandate. His cognition continues to decline gradually. Two years after the initial visit, he needs help with basic activities of daily living and is occasionally incontinent. He has home care services at home. His wife has taken over financial management, using the power of attorney. She has to watch him constantly as he falls easily, including falling off chairs and falling when he gets up at night to urinate. She rarely has a decent night's sleep. His MMSE score is 15/30.

Six months later, he is admitted to hospital with delirium. His wife says that she can no longer take care of him, and he is discharged to a nursing home, with his consent. His wife would like to sell the house, which is in his name, and move into a small apartment close to the nursing home.

Shortly after discharge, you receive a call from the patient's sister in Boston. She says that his wife should be caring for him at home and had no business sending him to the nursing home. She says she will go to court if necessary to have him sent home.

You see the patient to assess decision-making capacity. The patient believes that he can still drive and care for himself. He is not sure whether he has moved recently. He does not know what his income or expenses are. After a detailed examination you find him incapable of making personal decisions and managing his assets. His wife obtains a psychosocial assessment from their social worker, and their notary (who has a distinct legal role in Quebec) initiates the process to have the protection mandate homologated.

*****

Sound ethics requires that we not examine or treat any patient without having obtained their informed consent to do so. If a patient lacks the capacity to make an informed decision about treatment, a substitute decision-maker must be sought.

The terms **Competency, Decision-making capacity** and **Aptitude** are sometimes used interchangeably to reflect the same notion. We will use the term **Capacity** or **Decision-making capacity,** which is used widely in the medical literature.

Decision-making capacity is a person's ability to make, and act on, his or her own decisions.

Where do we start?

For a long time capacity was decided on the basis of diagnosis. This is sometimes called the **status approach.** A person who had a cognitive or psychiatric disorder was no longer allowed to make decisions. As our collective understanding of brain disorders improved, it became apparent that this black-and-white distinction lacked the necessary subtlety and unjustly categorized people. In the twentieth century, most jurisdictions updated their laws to require individual capacity evaluation before declaring anyone incapable.

It can also be tempting to base our opinion on the reasonableness of the decision being made by the person, typically a refusal of a medical treatment thought necessary: the **outcome approach**. A "**functional approach**" assesses whether a person's knowledge, skills and abilities allow her/ him to make a particular decision in a particular context. Now we commonly use an **integrated approach**, in which a patient's **status** (diagnosis) or foreseen **outcome** (decision-making that is seen as harmful) triggers a **functional** decision-making capacity assessment.

Criteria

There is a widely accepted consensus on four criteria to be used to decide whether a patient is capable of decision-making.[1] They could be summarized as follows:

- Ability to **understand** information relevant to decision-making;
- Ability to **appreciate** the significance of that information for one's own situation;
- Ability to **reason** with relevant information so as to engage in a logical process of weighing options;
- Ability to **express a choice.**

Someone who can **understand, appreciate, reason** and **express a choice** is capable of decision-making. Someone who lacks all these abilities is not. Of course they all admit of degrees, and a person may have lost some abilities but not others, whence the need to look at each pertinent decision in detail in order to fairly judge the patient's capacity.

The assessment

The fact that the determination of a person's capacity cannot be based on a diagnosis alone does not excuse us from knowing the diagnosis, either through our own examination or by information received from another physician. The situation might be very different depending on whether the patient has a possibly transient disorder such as delirium, a progressive disorder such as dementia, an intermittent and potentially treatable disorder such as psychosis or severe depression, or a fixed disorder such as a developmental disorder or head injury.

Prior to the assessment, it is important to have precise information on the reasons it is being requested. If such an assessment is not required for the patient's well-being or the safety of their property, it should not be done. We also need objective and detailed information about the decisions that need to be made and the alleged lack of judgment or reasoning ability. This allows us to evaluate the patient with respect to her own life and needs, rather than using abstract theoretical examples. For financial capacity we need objective information on the patient's financial situation.

We begin with brief cognitive testing. The Mini-Mental State Examination[2] is by no means an instrument to determine capacity, but the score can provide useful information. For example, one study[3] showed that incapacity is more likely in patients with a score below 19, and capacity more likely if the score is over 23. Psychiatric examination is also necessary, to determine if the patient has a mood disorder severe enough to affect decision-making (e.g. causing loss of hope, diminished self-worth), or psychosis relevant to the decision (e.g. "my doctor wants to harm me"). We then proceed to assess the patient's ability to **understand, appreciate, reason** and **express a choice**, as applied to the type of decision being questioned. We do so by "walking through" the decision with the patient.

Capacity to consent to medical treatment

Does the patient understand the nature of the illness, the nature and purpose of the proposed treatment, the benefits and risks of the proposed treatment, and alternative treatment options?

Does the patient appreciate how this information applies to his personal situation? Does he/she acknowledge the presence of the medical condition, and appreciate the expected consequences (**to him or herself**) of the proposed treatment and of the alternatives, including no treatment?

Is the patient able to reason, i.e. engage in a rational process of manipulating the relevant information? Can the patient express a choice and reasons for the choice? Does the patient consistently express the same choice? If so, the patient is capable of making the decision.

Several tools have been devised to help clinicians assess capacity to make medical decisions. A very helpful one is the **Aid to Capacity Evaluation**, from the University of Toronto.[4] It is essentially a structured interview to help answer the above questions.

Law courts across Canada frequently use the **Nova Scotia criteria**[5]:

"In determining whether or not a person in a hospital or a psychiatric facility is capable of consenting to treatment, the examining psychiatrist shall consider whether the person understands and appreciates: (a) the condition for which the specific treatment is proposed; (b) the nature and purpose of the specific treatment; (c) the risks and benefits involved in undergoing the specific treatment; and (d) the risks and benefits involved in not undergoing the specific treatment."

Capacity to make personal decisions (living situation)

Other personal decisions for which patients' capacity may be questioned often are related to their living situation: can they make capable decisions regarding the safety of living in their own home, or a possible need for help or supervision, or to move into a more structured environment? We apply the same criteria to the patient's approach to these decisions:

Does she/he **understand** any change of health status or circumstances that might affect the living situation; potential risks related to the living situation; and possible interventions to reduce the risk (get help, move, etc.)? Can he/she **appreciate** the effect of a change of health status or circumstances on his/her own safety or well-being in a given living situation; and the expected consequences of living with the risks, or of intervening? Is the patient able to reason, i.e. engage in a rational process of manipulating the relevant information? Can the patient express a choice and the reasons for the choice? Does the patient consistently express the same choice? If so, the patient is capable of making the decision.

Capacity to manage one's assets and make financial decisions

Managing one's financial affairs requires similar abilities to other decision-making: being able to understand, appreciate, reason and express a choice. It also requires certain skills.

Does the patient understand her/his financial situation; any problems there might be, related to financial management; changes in health or cognition that could make it difficult to manage finances; a possible need for help; and other decisions that need to be made? Can the patient appreciate the expected consequences of continuing as is, having help, having someone take over, of a possibly abusive situation, and of the various alternatives, in the case of other decisions? Is the patient able to reason, i.e. engage in a rational process of manipulating the relevant information? Can the patient express a choice? Express the reasons for the choice? Does the patient consistently express the same choice?

Does the patient possess sufficient functional skills to be able to manage his affairs independently? This might include receiving income and paying bills, banking, and budget management, or more complex skills such as making decisions about investments or other property. Are the patient's memory, ability to calculate and organizational abilities sufficient to continue carrying out these tasks? We should keep in mind how the patient organized these tasks in the past: has a meticulous record-keeper lost the ability to maintain and balance his/her chequebook? Or was his/her style always haphazard but good enough for his/her needs? A patient who can understand, appreciate, reason and express choices about financial issues, and has the necessary skills to carry out the financial management required by his own situation, is capable of continuing to do so.

Decision-making for patients with dementia

A patient with early dementia may retain capacity to make decisions in many spheres. We know, however, that the disease is likely to progress, and that decision-making capacity will be gradually lost. It is thus very important, at the time of diagnosis, to find out whether the patient has made plans for the future, and if not to encourage him/her to do so. This may include making a will, giving a power of attorney or protection mandate, and advance care planning.

When a patient with dementia lives alone, safety hazards may arise, such as fire risk, malnutrition, or the effects of forgetting essential medicines or taking them inappropriately. Many such patients lack insight into the presence of the dementia and assume they have normal cognition. Decisions based on this assumption are not competent decisions, and if the patient refuses interventions to improve his/her safety, steps must be taken to formally assess decision-making capacity and name a substitute decision-maker.

Conversely, some patients with early cognitive symptoms may retain insight and be able to address problems and even to competently accept certain risks in order to maintain their independence, thus entering into conflict with family members who want their safety at all costs.

Even when a person is clearly incapable of decision-making, fundamental respect for the person requires us to continue caring for him in keeping with her/his known values and wishes. This might include food preferences and special diets, maintaining his/her appearance and grooming, religious observance, as well as favourite routines and activities. An elder with dementia remains a full member of the human community and should be treated as such.

Capacity to sign legal documents

Power of attorney:
"You can give someone a power of attorney to represent you when you cannot do something yourself...."[6]

A bank or notary may request a letter from a doctor attesting to an older patient's capacity to give a power of attorney. To be capable, the patient must understand the concept and content of the document and its possible implications, including the approximate value of the assets, the power that is being entrusted, the risk of harm to the assets from poor judgment or dishonesty on the part of the mandatary, and the fact that she/he has the right to revoke the power of attorney at any time.

Protection mandate:
A protection mandate "is a document that lets you name, in advance, one or several people to look after your well-being and manage your property if you become incapable of doing this yourself."[7] It has no effect while the person who signed it remains capable of decision-making.

To be capable of signing a protection mandate, the patient must possess the same capacities as for a power of attorney. In addition, she/he must understand that the power given only takes effect if in the future she/he becomes incapable of decision-making, and that after that time it can no longer be revoked. She/he must understand that it applies not only to management of property but also to personal decisions such as health care or housing.

Testamentary capacity

To be capable of making a will, the patient must understand its nature and effect, and recollect approximately what property he/she has and the persons who might expect to inherit from him/her. He/she must understand the extent of what is being given to each beneficiary, and know if he/she has excluded someone who might have expected to benefit.

Protective supervision

Decision-making capacity only needs to be formally assessed if it is required for the protection of the person or her/his property. Many families continue to care for their loved ones and to manage their affairs without any such assessment. For example, they may continue to manage their assets online or using a power of attorney, and to make personal decisions in consultation with the patient. All adults are presumed capable unless there is evidence to the contrary.

"Under the law, the need for protection exists when an incapacitated person must be assisted or represented in the exercise of their civil rights. This need may arise from the person's isolation, the duration of their incapacity, the nature or state of the person's affairs, etc."[8]

We might need to assess capacity, for example, if there is disagreement among family members regarding the needs of the patient, or if major financial transactions are foreseen, such as the sale of a house. In cases of abuse or neglect, a legal decision-maker may be required to protect the person from harm. Finally, if the person refuses interventions essential for his/her safety, or has delusions regarding those caring for him/her, capacity assessment will be needed.

If a person who has become incapable of decision-making has a protection mandate, the family may proceed to have it homologated.[9] This requires a medical assessment and a psychosocial assessment by a social worker. Through a juridical process, the person is declared incapable and the mandatary named. This is usually undertaken by the family with the help of a notary or lawyer.

If there is no protection mandate, the family or another concerned party may apply for private or public curatorship or tutorship. If the person is only partially incapable a tutor is named, who is responsible for some decisions, while the patient retains control of others, as determined by the court. If totally incapable, a curator is named. Wherever possible, the tutor or curator will be a family member or friend of the patient. If no one is available, this role is taken by the Public Curator.[10]

Back to the case

When you first saw Don, he had early cognitive symptoms but still independent, and was presumed capable of making decisions. On your advice he put measures into place to authorize his wife to make personal and financial decisions in his name should he lose capacity. She was able to care for him for several years without any formal capacity assessment; it became necessary when a major financial transaction was being contemplated and a family member was challenging her authority to make decisions on his behalf. You found that Don lacked the necessary understanding, appreciation and ability to reason and express a choice about his personal and financial needs. Protective supervision was put into place.

1. Applebaum PS, Grisso T. Assessing patients' capacity to consent to treatment. NEJM 1988; 319:1635-1638
2. https://www.ncbi.nlm.nih.gov/pubmed/1202204
3. https://www.ncbi.nlm.nih.gov/pmc/articles/ PMC271553/
4. http://www/jcb.utoronto.ca/tools/documents/ documents/ace.pdf
5. Nova Scotia Hospitals Act article 52.sA: https:// nslegislature.ca/sites/default/files/legc/statutes/ hospital.pdf

6. https://www.educaloi.qc.ca/en/capsules/power-attorney

7. https://www.educaloi.qc.ca/en/capsules/protection-mandates-naming-someone-act-you

8. Ibid

9. https://www.educaloi.qc.ca/en/capsules/protection-mandates-naming-someone-act-you

10. http://www.curateur.gouv.qc/cura/en/majeur/inaptitude/role/index.html

HOW DO I PROTECT MY PATIENT?

Randy S. Perskin, Esq., JD,
Elder Law Attorney, New York

VIGNETTE

Mary Smith is a 75 year old woman with early onset dementia diagnosed by her physician. She is otherwise healthy and is able to perform ADLs (activities of daily living) such as toileting and bathing. She is married, lives with her husband, and has two adult children who care for her deeply.

As the dementia progresses Ms. Smith becomes confused and although she speaks clearly she cannot follow conversations or express her concerns. Although mobile, she needs direction for purposes of dressing, bathing, toileting and feeding herself. It is no longer safe for her to perform certain daily tasks unattended such as cooking. She can no longer travel outdoors without company as she will often forget where she is, where she is going or where she lives.

Ms. Smith, when suffering from advanced dementia, is not self directing. She becomes unable to coordinate her care and needs assistance with all activities of daily living to the extent that she needs reminders to take her medications, bathe and pay her bills. Although she is still physically healthy it is no longer safe for her to be left to her own devices.

DISCUSSION

Considerations in the care and treatment of the elder population focus on personal needs, including but not limited to healthcare, living situation, and property management. This latter includes payment of bills and managing finances. Elder adults who suffer from physical disabilities which do not impact on their ability to handle their needs or who do not suffer from any significant incapacity can continue to manage their needs as they always have. The issues facing elder persons who suffer from disabilities which impact their ability to understand their needs and manage them can be effectively dealt with if the proper safeguards are in place.

Advance Directives can protect the elder population if and when they can no longer care for themselves. Agents can be appointed to effectively stand in the place of the elder person to make decisions on their behalf should they be unable to do so. In the United States, the Health Insurance Portability and Accountability Act of 1996 (HIPAA) restricts the ability of health care providers and insurance companies to provide personal health information (PHI) without consent.[11] Although protecting a patient's privacy is of significant importance, concerns arise when an individual requires the support of others for care, management and treatment. Pursuant to Federal Law, a health care provider can discuss relevant health information and billing practices if either the patient gives consent, or with family members involved with the care, treatment and payment if in the provider's professional judgment the patient would consent.[12] That being said the patient can limit the amount of information given to family members. A HIPAA Release can be executed allowing the health care provider to release information to the named individual. The Family Health Care Decisions Act (FHCDA)[13] establishes the authority for health care providers in general hospitals and health care facilities, notably nursing homes, to speak with family members or close friends in order to make health care decisions should the patient become unable to do so. FHCDA can be applied when the elder person is in an institutional setting and healthcare decisions need to be made for a patient no longer able to act on their own behalf. However it does not apply to those individuals in the community who may need the assistance of others in making determinations on their own behalf. A Health Care Proxy can be executed, appointing an agent to act on an individual's behalf for purposes of medical care, including care management, in case of an inability to act.[14] An agent should act in accordance, as much as possible, with the principal's wishes even if they disagree. As such, the principal should have a conversation with their agent as to their wishes and desires regarding health care issues. The Health Care Proxy should indicate that the agent is aware of the principal's wishes in such regard. The preferences can be related orally or in writing. The Health Care Proxy will become effective when it is determined that the principal no longer has the capacity to act for him/herself.

A Living Will is a document that sets forth health care wishes regarding life prolonging procedures and other end of life care. A Living Will can specify the types of treatment desired to prolong life or the measures that the principal wishes to be avoided.

A Do Not Resuscitate Order (DNR), on the other hand, is generally written by doctors in a hospital and specifically instructs health care professionals not to perform CPR or other life sustaining measures when the heart beat or breathing stops.

A Power of Attorney is a legal document which appoints an agent to act with regard to financial and legal matters.[15] It can be as broad or as specific as desired and is often used to protect a party who is unable to act on their own behalf with regard to their financial needs. There are three types of Powers of Attorney: Nondurable, Durable and Springing. A Nondurable Power of Attorney usually applies to a specific transaction such as the sale of a home. A Nondurable Power of Attorney is valid until revoked or the principal becomes incapacitated. A Durable Power of Attorney allows an agent to act on behalf of the principal even after incapacity. A Durable Power of Attorney is often used to avoid unnecessary and expensive Guardianships. A Durable Power of Attorney can be revoked and is valid until the death of the principal. A Springing Power of Attorney becomes effective when a named event, such as the incapacity of the principal, arises or after a specified period of time. Generally for incapacity purposes a letter from a physician testifying to that circumstance will work. Powers of Attorney become effective when signed, except for a Springing Power of Attorney. However it is the intent of the Durable Power of Attorney that the agent will act once the principal becomes unable to do so. Effective September 2009 and further amended in September 2010 changes were made to the statutory short form Power of Attorney to the effect that the Power of Attorney must contain the signatures of both the principal and agent; the agent's authority to make gifts be granted through a separate statutory gifts rider that has the signatures of two witnesses; multiple agents must act together unless otherwise designated; a principal can appoint someone to monitor the actions of the agent: this person has the authority to request records of transactions entered into on behalf of the principal; the principal's rights are stated on the first page in bold faced print; the agent's role, fiduciary obligations and legal limitations are explained; and a signature constitutes acknowledgement. A Power of Attorney in New York can also include language allowing for the release of medical information protected under HIPAA for financial planning purposes, specifically the payment of medical bills. A Power of Attorney drafted prior to 2009, if compliant with the General Obligations Law, can remain in full force and effect. It is possible that a Power of Attorney can be accepted multi jurisdictionally if drafted in accordance with the General Obligations Law or the law of the state where it was executed. A conversation with an attorney well versed in the law in this regard is recommended.

Agents acting under a Power of Attorney are fiduciaries and should act in the best interests of the principal. Proper record keeping is imperative. Interested parties, such as financial institutions and family members, can bring special proceedings questioning the agent's actions. The appointment of an agent to act under a Power of Attorney is a decision which should not be taken lightly. The agent should be someone who the principal trusts and has an understanding of their financial situation and needs.

Practical issues in dealing with Advance Directives include capacity. It is hoped that proper planning is put into effect prior to the occurrence of incapacity. Capacity for purposes of executing the proper Advance Directives means the ability to understand the nature of the document being signed and the authority being granted. An attorney skilled in the preparation of such documents, either in conjunction with estate planning or separately, can effectively determine if such capacity exists. By interviewing the principal, asking questions about their wishes, explaining the documents and relating the issues therein, a reputable and knowledgeable attorney can make a determination as to the capacity for these purposes. Optimally, an attorney well versed in elder care issues is consulted. Essentially, a person with diagnoses that affect mental capacity, such as early onset dementia, may not be precluded from creating advance directives.

Even the most comprehensive Advance Directive will not be properly utilized if its existence is unknown. In this regard copies should be provided to any agents appointed, to medical and healthcare providers where necessary, to financial institutions and in the case of Health Care Proxies and Living Wills kept on hand on the principal's person, as in a wallet. Originals and copies should be kept somewhere safe but not necessarily in a safety deposit box which cannot be accessed by the appropriate parties. Discussions with family members, close personal friends or agents as to the existence of Advance Directives and their locations is important.

Under New York law there are two types of Guardianships that can be established. The Surrogates Court Procedure Act (SCPA) Article 17-A can be used to establish a Guardianship for people who are mentally retarded or developmentally disabled attributable to conditions such as cerebral palsy or neurological imbalances.[16] A Guardianship can be established for elderly persons, trauma victims and, at times, mentally ill or developmentally disabled persons pursuant to Article 81 of the Mental Hygiene Law.[17]

A Guardianship proceeding pursuant to Article 81 of the Mental Hygiene Law (MHL) is commenced by Order to Show Cause and Verified Petition in the county where the Alleged Incapacitated Person (AIP), the person to whom the Guardianship proceeding relates, resides or is physically present. The petitioner can be the AIP, the CEO of a facility in which the AIP is a resident, an adult relative, Adult Protective Services, or any other person concerned with the welfare of the AIP. The Order to Show Cause includes identification information for the AIP, such as name and address, as well as the reasons why a Guardianship is being sought. A Verified Petition is more detailed in that in addition to the information given in the Order to Show Cause it will include financial information, a description of the functional level of the AIP including behavior, understanding and appreciation of the nature and consequences of any inability to manage personal needs or property. Factual allegations of actual occurrences, demonstrating that the AIP will suffer harm due to her/his lack of understanding of the consequences of the inability to provide for personal needs or property management, are tailored to relate to the powers being sought, the duration of the powers being sought, and the approximate value and description of the financial assets of the AIP. It is noted whether the AIP is a recipient of public assistance, the nature of any claim, debt or obligation of the AIP, names addresses and telephone numbers of any presumptive distributes, available resources and an opinion as to the sufficiency of those resources as well as other information which would assist the Court Evaluator in conducting an investigation and writing a report.

There are instances where a Temporary Restraining Order is included in the Order to Show Cause, for example where there is an eviction proceeding pending or where abuse is alleged. Language to the effect that personal medical information may be provided should additionally be included in the Order to Show Cause. An AIP may consent to provide health care information protected by HIPAA, or a Court Evaluator can move to obtain a Court Order to obtain medical records. Additional Orders might be necessary where records from financial institutions are required.

Once the Order to Show Cause is signed by a Judge, a hearing date will be set within 28 days of the date of the Order. The Judge will generally appoint a Court Evaluator who is responsible for explaining the Guardianship proceeding to the AIP, investigating the claims made and writing a report, including recommendations, to be supplied to the Court. The report should also relate any jurisdictional and service issues. The report may also be supplied to the attorney for the AIP and Petitioner with prior Court approval.

The Court Evaluator is an independent individual appointed by the Court to effectively act as the eyes and ears of the Court and does not represent any of the parties in the Guardianship proceeding. The Court Evaluator does not have to be an attorney. An attorney for the AIP can also be appointed for representation in the Guardianship proceeding. The attorney for the AIP acts as an advocate. Personal service of the Order to Show Cause and Petition, as well as the Notice of Proceeding which sets forth the time date and place of the hearing, is required. Service of the Order to Show Cause, Verified Petition and Notice of Proceeding should also be effectuated on the Court Evaluator and attorney for the AIP. Service of the Order to Show Cause and Notice of Proceeding, not the Verified Petition, should additionally be effectuated on other interested parties such as the spouse, adult children, siblings and the person with whom the AIP resides.

The AIP is entitled to be present at the Hearing. The AIP's appearance can be waived if it is determined that they cannot meaningfully participate. Generally, the Court will make every effort to allow for the AIP's participation including adjourning the hearing where necessary or conducting bedside hearings. At the Hearing evidence will be presented via testimony, including that of the Court Evaluator, a psychiatric care provider if a psychological assessment was provided, the AIP, as well as family members and other interested parties if available and relevant. Documentary evidence, such as the Court Evaluator's report is introduced into the record. After listening to the testimony and reviewing the evidence the judge will make a determination as to the Guardianship.

The Court's determination as to the Guardianship will be set forth in an Order and Judgment. The Court, in making its determination, should consider the least restrictive alternative thereby giving the AIP the greatest amount of freedom while considering functional limitations that make it difficult to understand or appreciate the nature or consequences of any inability to provide for personal needs or property management. The desires of the AIP are therefore taken into account. The Guardianship can be tailored to the specific needs of the AIP and be broad or narrow. Primary consideration is given to family members, however independent Guardians are often appointed particularly where there are allegations of abuse or neglect, where there is no family member available or where a particular skill set is required to resolve particular issues.

The AIP may be declared an Incapacitated Person, within the scope of Article 81 of the Mental Hygiene Law. It is significant that incapacity in this regard is a legal, not medical, term and limits an individual's ability to enter into contracts or other legal issues that require capacity. However it is not always the case that a person is adjudged incapacitated for purposes of a Guardianship. There are instances where an individual is designated as a Person in Need of a Guardian (PING) usually for specific issues that need to be addressed by a Guardian.

A Guardian can be appointed for personal needs or property management. A Guardian of the Person can be given powers that relate to personal needs such as determining the living situation, health care and placement of aides. A Guardian of the Property can be given powers relating to property management including marshalling and managing assets, paying bills and applying for and maintaining private and public benefits. A Guardianship can be tailored to the specific needs of the AIP. Therefore a Guardian's powers can be limited to a specific issue, such as dealing with an eviction proceeding and relocations issues, stopping abuse, or Medicaid planning. Additionally a Guardian of the Property may be appointed but not a Guardian of the Person. A Temporary Guardian may be appointed during the pendency of the proceeding in order to assist with specific issues that need immediate attention. A Guardian, once appointed, will have the powers set forth in the Order and Judgment upon obtaining a commission to act. If an expansion of powers is necessary an order can be obtained via motion for such purposes. The Guardianship terminates upon the death of the IP or PING or the completion of the duties set forth in the Order and Judgment.

Guardianships are subject to Court oversight. A Guardian is required to submit an Initial Report within 90 days of appointment detailing the ward's current circumstances, and Annual Accounting thereafter. Annual Accountings will be reviewed by a Court Examiner appointed by the Court and a report and proposed order to judicially settle the account will be presented to the Court. Upon the death of the ward, following notice to the Court, a Final Accounting can be presented which can be reviewed by a Referee to Review for purposes of settling the Final Account and discharge. In instances of Temporary or Limited (Special) Guardianships a Report will generally be submitted describing the actions taken to resolve the issues addressed in the Order and Judgment.

Guardianship fees, to the Court Evaluator, Attorney for the AIP and on occasion to the petitioning attorney can be chargeable to the AIP's estate. Additionally, payment to the appointed Guardian is also generally made from the ward's funds. Where limited funds are available fees are often paid by the Department of Social Services to the Court Evaluator or Temporary Guardian and to the attorney for the AIP.

A Guardianship can be transferred to another state pursuant to the Uniform Adult Guardianship and Protective Proceeding Act (UAGPPJA) when adopted by that state. Such a transfer can alleviate the expense and duplicative work required to establish a new Guardianship in a different state. Discussions with an attorney familiar with the UAGPPJA and the states that have adopted it should be entered into when such a transfer may be necessary.

Practical considerations for the aging population include safe living arrangements and financial management. A Geriatric Care Manager, usually a trained nurse or social worker, can assist in determining the specific needs of the elder client and locate housing and other services that are appropriate for care. Various factors need to be considered in determining whether the elder person should remain at home or consider placement in a nursing home or assisted living facility. In determining whether it is safe for an elder adult to live in the community, the condition of the home should be considered, whether assistance is needed to provide for the activities of daily living and whether the individual lives alone or with someone else who can be responsible for their care. Health aides are an invaluable resource to an elder individual who is no longer totally independent but wishes to reside at home. Assisted living facilities and nursing homes are alternatives to a community residence when an elder individual needs more care than can be safely provided in the home. A nursing home generally follows more of a medical model than assisted living facilities do. Assisted living communities therefore provide more of a home atmosphere. Many assisted living facilities in New York do not accept Medicaid or Medicare so financial concerns can come into play.

Financial planning for the elder population includes determining if they are receiving the benefits they need to survive. Long term care insurance is a private policy that covers the expenses for assistance in the community with the activities of daily living, and health aides. The cost of long term care insurance depends on the age at which it was purchased. Medicare parts A, hospital, and B, medical, is available to any person in any state upon reaching age 65. Medicare Part D, for prescription drug coverage, can be obtained through any Medicare approved insurance carrier. Supplemental insurance can be used to cover those expenses that Medicare does not, such as copays. Medicaid is a needs based program for low income families. The income and asset levels vary from state to state. In New York, community Medicaid can be used to pay for health aides, in addition to healthcare, and institutional Medicaid can be used to pay for nursing homes. Medicaid rules and qualification issues are complicated and the proper planning should be discussed with an elder law attorney expert in the field. Social security retirement benefits in New York can be collected at age 62. A Representative Payee is an individual who is determined to be qualified to collect social security benefits for the senior individual. Supplemental Security Income, SSI, is a federal income supplement program designed to help aged blind and disabled people who have little or no income and is used to meet basic needs such as food, shelter and clothing. Social Security Disability, SSD, is a federal program designed to supplement the income of people whose physical disabilities limit their ability to work. The Supplemental Nutrition Assistance program, SNAP, is a federal income supplement program designed to assist people in obtaining food, previously recognized as food stamps. The Senior Citizens Rent Increase Exemption, SCRIE, freezes the rent of head of households aged 62 and older who live in rent regulated apartments in New York City. Death benefits from a spouse, either from social security or pensions, should also be explored.

Recognizing the signs of elder abuse in the aged population is a key factor in their care. Elder abuse, which can be physical, financial or psychological, may occur at the hands of a caregiver or other person in a position of trust. See the chapter on Elder Abuse for further information.

Financial exploitation can include the misuse of funds or the taking of property. Financial abuse can be recognized by a financial institution if funds are withdrawn without the consent of the account holder or their representative. Additionally, there have been instances where caretakers take their aged clients to the bank to withdraw cash for them or simply use their bank card. In such instances a financial representative can step in to protect the interests of the elder client. Physical and psychological abuse cannot be as easily identified especially where the elder person has a disability that prevents him from communicating what is happening. Physical injuries can be the result of abuse. If the injury resulted from someone pushing or hitting the senior it qualifies as abuse. If the elder person lives in an assisted living community or nursing home there are often cameras set up in the hallways and public areas thereby giving proof positive of abusive behavior. Additionally, such institutions are highly regulated. An incidence report should be generated detailing the incident and steps that were taken to prevent it from happening again. Abuse can take the form of neglect, even self inflicted in the case of an individual who is not properly feeding themselves or obtaining the proper medical treatment. Such incidences can be reported to Adult Protective Services (APS) who can then step in and evaluate whether protection needs to be implemented and the form it should take. The Attorney General of the State of New York has an elder abuse hotline where instances of abuse can be reported. Complaints are investigated and it is then determined whether the incidence rises to the level of a criminal act. The Elder Abuse Education and Outreach Program provides information and advice to elder abuse victims and their caregivers. Even if an act does not rise to the level of elder abuse it still may be negligent, such as in the case where no care or inappropriate care is given for an injury. In such cases a civil action may be brought and discussions with a personal injury attorney can be useful.

It should be noted that all references herein are made to New York Law unless otherwise indicated as Federal Law of the United States. Advice of counsel in the jurisdiction of residence should be used to navigate the legal ramifications of the needs of an elderly client.

CONCLUSION

Mrs. Smith's son consulted counsel when his mother was originally diagnosed with dementia. He was asked whether she had any Advance Directives in place. As he was uncertain, he was advised to see if his mother had a Will, as often Advance Directives are put in place when estate planning is performed. Fortunately Mrs. Smith was able to remember the name of the attorney who prepared her Will. It was discovered that Advance Directives, including a Power of Attorney and Health Care Proxy, had been executed and were effectively used to assist Mrs. Smith when she became unable to manage her finances and personal needs. It was fortuitous that Mrs. Smith had a loving family that was able to work together to protect her interests.

*Disclaimer: The information contained in this chapter is provided only as general information and not intended as legal advice, nor should it be used as a substitute for complete review of your case by an experienced elder law attorney. All situations differ. By reading this chapter there is no attorney client relation established between you and Randy S. Perskin, Esq.

11. 1. HIPAA; PUBL 104-191, 110 flat 1936.
12. 45 CFR 164.510(b)
13. Public Health Law Articles 29-CC & 29-CCC
14. Public Health law Article 29-C
15. General Obligations Law Section 5-1501
16. Surrogates Court Procedures Act Article 17-A
17. Mental Hygiene Law Article 81

GLOSSARY

The Care of the Older Person

Medical and Scientific Terms and their Meanings:
- **Chapter references** refer to: **The Care of the Older Person**
- **Page references** refer to: **Long Life: A Survival Strategy**; Ronald M Caplan 2008 www.livinglonger.wordpress.com Click: **Manuscript** (ID: rcaplanmd) Password: source
- **www.rcaplanmd.com : Bibliography**

ACCOUNTABLE CARE ORGANIZATION (ACO): Medical provider organization that incentivizes cost and quality control, for example by reducing inpatient utilization and specialist referrals. Includes **Medicare Shared Savings Program (MSSP),** which sets a target cost of care for patients.

ACE INHIBITOR: Drug that inhibits the angiotensin-converting enzyme, stopping the formation of Angiotensin II which constricts blood vessels. Blood pressure is lowered, because blood vessels are opened up, and blood can flow more freely. P.75
http://www.medicinenet.com/ace_inhibitors/article.htm

ACETYLCHOLINE: A neurotransmitter. P.177, 382
http://www.ncbi.nlm.nih.gov/books/NBK11143/

ACNE: Chronic skin condition characterized by seborrhea (oily secretion) and blocked follicles (comedomes) including blackheads and whiteheads that may become infected. P.391, 393
https://online.epocrates.com/diseases/10111/Acne-vulgaris/Key-Highlights

ACRYLAMIDE: Chemical that can form during high heat food preparation of high starch foods from the amino acid asparagine in combination with some sugars. Possible carcinogen in high doses. P.283
https://www.cancer.gov/about-cancer/causes-prevention/risk/diet/acrylamide-fact-sheet

ADDICTION: Physiologic compulsive need for a substance, use of that substance, inability to abstain, development of tolerance to it, and distinctive withdrawal symptoms and signs. See "**Opioid**". P.9, 330
https://www.cdc.gov/drugoverdose/index.html

ADHESION: Abnormal union of surfaces, or fibrous tissue bands between structures. P.250
https://www.ncbi.nlm.nih.gov/pmc/articles/PMC5295619/

ADOPTIVE CELL TRANSFER (ACT): Use of **Tumor-Infiltrating Lymphocytes (TILs)** to overcome immunosuppressive signals and eradicate cancer cells.
https://www.cancer.gov/about-cancer/treatment/types/immunotherapy

ADVANCE DIRECTIVE: Legal document that ensures one's wishes are followed in the event a person cannot make their own decisions. See: The Care of the Older Person: How do I protect my patient? : Randy S. Perskin

https://ag.ny.gov/sites/default/files/advancedirectives.pdf

AGING: Gradual loss of physiological functions accompanied by increasing risk of mortality and decreasing fertility. See: The Care of the Older Person: Introduction: Jose Morais
http://journal.frontiersin.org/article/10.3389/fgene.2016.00119/full
https://www.nature.com/articles/s41551-017-0093?WT.mc_id=EMI_NBME_1707_JULYISSUE_PORTFOLIO&spMailingID=54556746&spUserID=MTc3MDI4

ODk5NQS2&spJobID=1203835636&spReportId=
MTIwMzgzNTYzNgS2

AGONIST: Exogenous substance that goes to a cell receptor and produces a response. P.180
https://en.wikipedia.org/wiki/Agonist

AIDS: Autoimmune Deficiency Syndrome: Sexually transmitted infection caused by Human Immunodeficiency Viruses HIV-1 and HIV-2 which compromise the immune system. P.XIII, XVI, 31, 261, 262, 263
https://www.aids.gov/
http://www.thelancet.com/journals/lancet/article/PIIS0140-6736(14)60164-1/fulltext https://jamanetwork.com/journals/jama/article-abstract/2678246?utm source=silverchair&utm medium=email&utm campaign=article alert-jama&utm content=

ALBUMIN: Water soluble single chain protein synthesized in liver. Present in egg white and blood serum.
http://albumin.org/properties-of-human-serum-albumin-and-albumin-atomic-coordinates/

ALDOSTERONE: Mineralocorticoid hormone from adrenal cortex. Increases blood pressure. Implication in alopecia. P.392
https://en.wikipedia.org/wiki/Aldosterone

ALKALINE PHOSPHATASE: Immune protein enzymes that catalyze the hydrolysis of phosphate groups, freeing

inorganic phosphate.
http://journal.frontiersin.org/article/10.3389/
fimmu.2017.00897/full?utm_source=F-AAE&utm_
medium=EMLF&utm_campaign=MRK_352999_35_
Immuno_20170808_arts_A

ALLELE: One of the two forms of a gene, derived from either the mother or the father. Genes are carried on chromosomes. Chromosomes are paired, with one chromosome in each pair coming from the father, and one coming from the mother.
http://mcat-review.org/genetics.php

ALLOGRAFT: Transplant from human donor to genetically nonidentical human recipient. P.252
http://ndt.oxfordjournals.org/content/early/2013/04/25/ndt.gft087.full.pdf

ALOPECIA: Baldness P.391
https://www.ncbi.nlm.nih.gov/pmc/articles/PMC3149477/

ALZHEIMER'S DISEASE: AD. Common form of dementia. One characteristic is amyloid plaque deposition in the brain. P.173, 266, 298. See: The Care of the Older Patient: Doctor, My Wife Is Getting Forgetful: Serge Gauthier; Why Does My Patient Have Gait And Balance Disorders ? : Olivier Beauchet ; Incontinence In Older Adults: Samer Shamout, Lysanne Campeau

http://www.thelancet.com/journals/laneur/article/
PIIS1474-4422(16)00062-4/abstract
http://www.ncbi.nlm.nih.gov/pubmed/24028956
http://www.nature.com/nature/journal/v537/n7618/full
/537036a.html?WT.feed_name=subjects_neuroscience
http://www.jwatch.org/na42506/2016/10/06/new-bio-
logic-treatment-dramatically-shrinks-plaques
https://www.ncbi.nlm.nih.gov/pubmed/27025652
http://www.nature.com/neuro/multimedia/alzheimers/
index.html?WT.mc_id=BAN_NN_1612_Alzheimers
www.nature.com/neuro/multimedia/alzheimers/index.
html?WT.mc_id=TOC_NN_1216_Alzheimers&spMailin-
gID=54002625&spUserID=MTc2NTUxNjM5NAS2&
spJobID=1160

AMINO ACIDS: The building blocks of protein. Some
amino acids can be synthesized in the human body.
Essential amino acids must be supplied in the diet, as
they cannot be synthesized in the human body. P.38
http://www.biology.arizona.edu/biochemistry/problem_
sets/aa/aa.html

AMNIOTIC FLUID: The fluid surrounding the developing fetus, contained in the amniotic sac. The thin amniotic membrane is closely applied to the inner walls of the
uterus. P. VIII, 48
http://iaimjournal.com/wp-content/uploads/2014/11/9-
Amniotic-fluid-derived-stem-cells.pdf

AMYLOID: Beta amyloid. Protein fragments that can clump in amorphous plaques in degenerative disease. P. 177

https://www.nia.nih.gov/alzheimers/publication/part-2-what-happens-brain-ad/hallmarks-ad
http://www.nature.com/nature/journal/v537/n7618/full/nature19323.html

ANASTOMOSIS: Relinking of a tubular structure so that the lumen is patent. P. 246
http://plasticsurgery.stanford.edu/education/microsurgery/intraoperative.html

ANDROGEN: The "male" sex hormones. Present in women in different amounts than in males. In men, the testicles are the main source of androgens. In women, androgens are mainly derived from the adrenal glands that sit atop the kidneys, and from the ovaries. P. 109, 204, 244

https://www.britannica.com/science/androgen https://www.frontiersin.org/articles/10.3389/fimmu.2018.00794/full?utm source=F-AAE&utm medium=EMLF&utm campaign=MRK 632947 35 Immuno 20180508 arts A

ANDROGEN RECEPTOR ANTAGONISTS: Drugs that competitively inhibit testosterone from binding to prostate cancer cells.
http://www.nejm.org/doi/full/10.1056/NEJMra1701695?query=main_nav_lg

http://www.nejm.org/doi/full/10.1056/NEJMoa1715546?
query=main_nav_lg

ANDROSTENEDIONE: A form of androgen. P. 204,
244, 391
https://pubchem.ncbi.nlm.nih.gov/compound/andro-
stenedione#section=Top

ANEMIA: Deficiency of red blood cells or hemoglobin.
P. 329
https://www.jwatch.org/na45561/2017/11/29/
anemia-elderly-review?query=etoc_jwgenmed&
jwd=000012066693&jspc=OBG

ANEURYSM: Weakening in a blood vessel wall, leading
to a bulge. P. 86
http://stroke.ahajournals.org/content/44/12/3613
https://journals.lww.com/cardiologyinreview/Abstract
/2016/03000/Abdominal_Aortic_Aneurysms_and_Risk_
Factors_for.5.aspx

ANGINA (PECTORIS): Chest pain caused by inadequate
oxygenation (ischemia) of , and circulation to heart muscle, secondary to arteriosclerotic disease in the coronary
arteries which supply the heart. P. 65
https://emedicine.medscape.com/article
/150215-overview

ANGIOGENESIS: New blood vessel formation. P.43
http://www.nature.com/nrd/journal/v3/n5/full/
nrd1381.html

ANGIOGRAPHY: Radiologic visualization of blood vessels after injecting them with radiopaque dye. P.80
https://emedicine.medscape.com/article
/1603072-overview

ANGIOPLASTY: The opening of a narrowed blood vessel by balloon inflation, along with stent placement to preserve patency. P.83, 86
http://www.ncbi.nlm.nih.gov/pubmedhealth/
PMH0021296/

ANGIOTENSIN: A vasoconstricting hormone. Stimulates aldosterone release from the adrenal cortex. P. 76
http://www.ncbi.nlm.nih.gov/pubmed/8583476

ANGIOTENSIN RECEPTOR BLOCKER: ARB. Drug that blocks the angiotensin receptor. P. 76
http://www.ncbi.nlm.nih.gov/pmc/articles/PMC4395832
/

ANOREXIA: Eating disorder with self starvation and marked weight loss. The Care of the Older Person: Could My Patient Be Malnourished ?: Jose Morais. P. 55
https://jeatdisord.biomedcentral.com/articles/10.1186/
s40337-015-0040-8

ANTHRAX: Serious bacterial infection caused by Bacillus Anthracis. Can be acquired cutaneously, and via the respiratory and gastrointestinal tracts. P. 268
https://www.cdc.gov/anthrax/specificgroups/health-care-providers/index.html

ANTIBIOTIC: A drug that kills or inactivates bacteria. Often works by binding and disrupting bacterial ribosomes (see "Ribosome")
http://www.nature.com/nrmicro/journal/v13/n1/full/nrmicro3380.html
http://www.nature.com/ja/journal/v67/n1/full/ja201349a.html
https://en.wikipedia.org/wiki/List_of_antibiotics
http://mdlinx.pdr.net/pharma-news/news-article.cfm/6885214/antibiotic-resistant-bacteria-star-shaped-peptide

ANTIBODY: A substance that reacts with a foreign invader (antigen) inactivating it. P. 101, 253, 254
https://www.ncbi.nlm.nih.gov/pmc/articles/PMC4284445/
http://www.nature.com/milestones/mileantibodies/timeline/index.html

ANTIBODY-DRUG CONJUGATES: Antibodies linked to a toxic substance, such as radioactive material, bacterial product, or chemical.
https://www.ncbi.nlm.nih.gov/pubmed/27299281

https://www.ncbi.nlm.nih.gov/pubmed/26589413
https://www.ncbi.nlm.nih.gov/pubmed/24423619

ANTIGEN: Foreign invader of the body. P.253, 330
http://www.annualreviews.org/doi/abs/10.1146/
annurev-immunol-032712-095910

ANTIMETABOLITE: Substance that interferes with cell
metabolism by inhibiting or replacing a normal metabo-
lite. Used as chemotherapeutic agents in cancer. P. 167
http://www.ncbi.nlm.nih.gov/pubmed/23361267
http://www.slideshare.net/OribaDanLangoya/
antimetabolites-in-cancer-chemotherapy-23606975

ANTIMULLERIAN HORMONE: Produced by ovarian
granulosa cells. Prevents the depletion of follicles in the
ovary. P. 192
http://www.ncbi.nlm.nih.gov/pubmed/22646322

ANTIOXIDANT: Substance that prevents the chemical
combination of oxygen with various other substances,
such as fats. P. 290, 300
http://dspace.uni.lodz.pl:8080/xmlui/bitstream/handle
/11089/17754/bartosz2.pdf?sequence=1&isAllowed=y

ANTISENSE TECHNOLOGY: Turning off genes by
introducing pieces of the genetic code. P. 105
http://smart-therapeutics.com/Technology/
RNAi-Antisense-Technologyb

ANXIETY: Feeling of unease that can rise to the level of panic attacks. P. 218, 332

http://www.ajgponline.org/article/S1064-7481(16)30147-6 /abstract

AORTA: The main artery from the heart to other parts of the body.

http://teachmeanatomy.info/abdomen/vasculature/ arteries/aorta/

APHERESIS: Removing blood from the body for the purpose of eliminating a specific component, then reintroducing the blood into the body.

https://health.ucsd.edu/specialties/apheresis/ Documents/2011%20Conventional-apheresis-therapies. pdf

APOLIPOPROTEIN E (ApoE): Protein involved in fat metabolism. A variant is a disease risk factor. P.321

http://www.ncbi.nlm.nih.gov/pubmed/11882522

http://www.ncbi.nlm.nih.gov/pubmed/16432152

APOPTOSIS: Programmed cell death P. 18, 300

http://www.ncbi.nlm.nih.gov/pmc/articles/PMC2117903 /

https://www.ncbi.nlm.nih.gov/books/NBK26873/

http://journal.frontiersin.org/article/10.3389/ fimmu.2017.00961/full?utm_source=F-AAE&utm_ medium=EMLF&utm_campaign=MRK_368025_35_

Immuno_20170822_arts_A
https://www.frontiersin.org/articles/10.3389/
fimmu.2018.00241/full?utm_source=F-AAE&utm_
medium=EMLF&utm_campaign=MRK_571163_35_I

APPENDICITIS: Inflammation of the appendix. Can
be treated by minimally invasive surgery. Incidence has
possibly been lowered with antibiotic use. P.268, 269
http://www.bmj.com/content/357/bmj.j1703.full

APTAMER: Single stranded DNA or RNA molecule that
can bind to preselected targets
http://www.basepairbio.com/research-and-publications/
what-is-an-aptamer-2/

AROMATASE INHIBITORS: The enzyme aromatase
catalyzes conversion of testosterone to estradiol.
Aromatase inhibitors are drugs that prevent this type of
estradiol formation.
http://www.nature.com/nrc/journal/v15/n5/abs/
nrc3920.html
http://erc.endocrinology-journals.org/content/20/4/
R183.full

ARRHYTHMIA: (Cardiac) Abnormal beating of the
heart. Includes tachycardia (abnormally fast heartbeat),
bradycardia (abnormally slow heartbeat) and irregular
heartbeats.

http://www.clevelandclinicmeded.com/medicalpubs/
diseasemanagement/cardiology/cardiac-arrhythmias/

ART: Advanced **A**ssisted **R**eproductive Technology.
Techniques that enhance the ability to conceive children,
including ovum and sperm retrieval, and ICSI. P.246,
248

http://www.cdc.gov/reproductivehealth/infertility/
http://www.hfea.gov.uk/ICSI.html

ARTERIOSCLEROSIS: Literal meaning is hardening of
the arteries. In **atherosclerosis**, a common type, calcified
fat deposits build up in the lining of arteries, narrowing
and obstructing them. P.63, 67, 68, 69, 72, 99, 155, 157, 266,
298, 331.

http://www.ncbi.nlm.nih.gov/pubmed/11001066
http://bmcmedicine.biomedcentral.com/articles/10.1186
/1741-7015-11-117

ARTERY: A blood vessel that usually carries oxygenated blood from the heart to other areas of the body.
Exceptions are the pulmonary artery, which carries
blood from the heart to the lungs for oxygenation, and
the umbilical arteries in the fetus, which carry blood
from the fetus to the placenta for oxygenation. P.63
https://training.seer.cancer.gov/anatomy/cardiovascular
/blood/classification.html

ARTHRITIS: A group of conditions of varying etiology characterized by inflammation in the joints. P.163, 266, 314

http://www.rheumatology.org/Practice-Quality/Clinical-Support/Criteria/ACR-Endorsed-Criteria

ARTHROSCOPY: Direct visualization into the joints by minimally invasive technique. P.166

http://www.arthroscopytechniques.org/

http://www.bmj.com/content/357/bmj.j1982

ARTIFICIAL HEART: Mechanical device that replaces the heart. **Mechanical Cardiac Support** refers to devices that assist the failing heart. P.72

http://www.jhltonline.org/article/S1053-2498(14)00976-0/abstract

ASBESTOS: A mined mineral once widely used for insulation and fireproofing. Fibers can be released into the air which can be responsible for asbestosis, a serious lung disease. P.357

http://www.ncbi.nlm.nih.gov/pubmed/25444537

ATHEROSCLEROSIS: See "Arteriosclerosis"

http://www.atherosclerosis-journal.com/

ATP: Adenosine **T**ri**p**hosphate: A nucleotide involved in intracellular energy transfer. P.36

https://pubchem.ncbi.nlm.nih.gov/compound/Adenosine_triphosphate

ATROPHY: Wasting of body tissue. **SARCOPENIA** is the loss of skeletal muscle mass and function. **CACHEXIA,** which incorporates sarcopenia, is a complex metabolic wasting syndrome associated with underlying disease, characterized by unwanted weight loss, muscle atrophy, fatigue, weakness, and loss of appetite. P.201

https://www.ncbi.nlm.nih.gov/pubmed/22773188

https://www.ncbi.nlm.nih.gov/pmc/articles/
PMC3940510/

https://www.ncbi.nlm.nih.gov/pubmed/20886766

https://www.ncbi.nlm.nih.gov/pmc/articles/
PMC4269139/

https://www.ncbi.nlm.nih.gov/pmc/articles/
PMC3117995/

AURA: A perceptual disturbance. P.196

http://www.medicinenet.com/script/main/art.asp?
articlekey=2395

AUTOANTIBODY: Immune protein (mainly IgM) produced by the immune system that is directed against (targets) an individual's own proteins, tissues, or organs

https://www.ncbi.nlm.nih.gov/pmc/articles/
PMC2703183/

http://journal.frontiersin.org/article/10.3389/
fimmu.2017.00603/full?utm_source=F-AAE&utm_

medium=EMLF&utm_campaign=MRK_294450_35_
Immuno_20170608_arts_A

AUTOIMMUNE DISEASES: Diseases in which the
immune response is inappropriately triggered and
attacks the individual's own tissues and organs. Includes
systemic lupus erythematosus, rheumatoid arthritis,
multiple sclerosis and Sjogren's syndrome.
http://www.nature.com/nm/journal/v21/n7/full/
nm.3897.html
http://journal.frontiersin.org/article/10.3389/
fimmu.2016.00587/full?utm_source=newsletter&utm_
medium=email&utm_campaign=Immunology-w52-2016
http://www.clevelandclinicmeded.com/medicalpubs/
diseasemanagement/rheumatology/laboratory-evalua-
tion-rheumatic-diseases/
https://www.ncbi.nlm.nih.gov/pmc/articles/
PMC4122257/

AUTOPHAGY: Intracellular degradation delivering
cytoplasmic constituents to the lysosome. May have
implications in anti-aging and starvation adaptation.
http://genesdev.cshlp.org/content/21/22/2861.long
http://journal.frontiersin.org/article/10.3389/
fimmu.2016.00657/full?utm_source=newsletter&utm_
medium=email&utm_campaign=Immunology-w1-2017

BABY SHAKING SYNDROME: Abusive head trauma.
Brain tissue injury, as well as hemorrhage and edema,

may result. P.260
https://emedicine.medscape.com/article
/1176849-overview

BACTERIUM: (Pleural: Bacteria) An old name for a microscopic organism that can be present in, or invade, humans. A pathogenic bacterium , or microorganism is one that causes disease.
http://www.bode-science-center.com/center/relevant-pathogens-from-a-z.html

BARIATRIC (METABOLIC) SURGERY: Weight loss surgery for selected Type 2 Diabetics and obese patients. Includes gastric binding, stomach stapling, gastric bypass, and stomach shortening sleeve gastrectomy.
https://asmbs.org/patients/bariatric-surgery-procedures

BASAL GANGLIA: Region at the base of the brain with clusters of neurons including the caudate nucleus, putamen, and globus pallidus. P. 179
http://webspace.ship.edu/cgboer/basalganglia.html

BASE PAIR: Two (out of four) **nucleic acid bases** on a rung of the spiral ladder of **DNA**. The four nucleic acids involved are adenine (**A**), cytosine (**C**), guanine (**G**), and thymine (**T**). They code the sequences of amino acids that, in turn, make up the proteins. P.33
http://www.dictionary.com/browse/base-pair

BETA BLOCKER: A drug that lowers blood pressure by taking up the receptor sites that control blood pressure. P.66, 75

http://www.medicinenet.com/beta_blockers/article.htm

BETA CAROTENE: An antioxidant. Precursor of Vitamin A. P.300

http://www.medicalnewstoday.com/articles/252758.php

BILE ACID SEQUESTRANT: Drug that binds bile acids in the intestine, so that they are excreted. P.80

http://www.medicinenet.com/bile_acid_sequestrants/article.htm

BIOENGINEERING: Rearranging DNA. Manufacturing recombinant DNA. P.33, 39

http://www.mdpi.com/journal/bioengineering

BIOFEEDBACK: Training to acquire voluntary control of a body function, such as heart rate. P.358

http://www.ncbi.nlm.nih.gov/pubmedhealth/PMH0070200/

BIORHYTHM: Cyclic pattern of activity; recurring biologic process. P.291, 320. See **Circadian Rhythm**

BIOSIMILAR: Product that is highly similar to an approved biologic product

http://www.fda.gov/Drugs/DevelopmentApprovalProcess/

HowDrugsareDevelopedandApproved/
ApprovalApplications/TherapeuticBiologicApplications/
Biosimilars/default.htm
http://jamanetwork.com/journals/jama/fullarticle
/2590051
http://jamanetwork.com/journals/jama/article-abstract
/2590049

BISPHOSPHONATES: Class of drugs that prevent loss
of bone mass by inhibiting bone resorption by blocking
osteoclasts. P.209, 327
http://www.bmj.com/content/351/bmj.h3783

BLEPHAROPLASTY: Cosmetic eyelid surgery. P.380
https://www.ncbi.nlm.nih.gov/pmc/articles/
PMC2840922/

BLOCKCHAIN TECHNOLOGY in HEALTHCARE:
Interoperable platform that memorializes every event or
step ("Block") in a data stream, or chain. Implications in
personalized medicine, research, and appropriate healthcare data sharing with enhanced security.
http://bulletin.facs.org/2017/12/blockchain-technology-
in-health-care-a-primer-for-surgeons/#.WlezLK6nHX4

BODY MASS INDEX: BMI. A calculation of body fat.
Weight (kilograms) divided by height (meters squared).
The Care of the Older Person: Could My Patient Be
Malnourished? : Jose Morais

BONE DENSITY: Measurement of Calcium and other minerals in bone. P.200

http://www.ncbi.nlm.nih.gov/pmc/articles/PMC2685234/

BONE DENSITY SCAN: Low exposure Xray to measure bone density. P.200, 208

https://www.bones.nih.gov/health-info/bone/bone-health/bone-mass-measurement-what-numbers-mean

BONE SCAN: NUCLEAR: Imaging bone after radiotracer uptake to identify tumors, usually metastatic. P.98

https://www.ncbi.nlm.nih.gov/pmc/articles/PMC4553252/

BOTOX: Botulinum **tox**in type A. Inhibits acetylcholine release. P.382

http://www.ncbi.nlm.nih.gov/pmc/articles/PMC2856357/

BRCA GENES: Breast Cancer Genes 1 and 2. Inherited mutations that predispose to breast and ovarian cancer. BRCA1 may increase risk of endometrial cancer as well. P.XIII

http://oncology.jamanetwork.com/article.aspx?articleid=2531470

https://www.sgo.org/wp-content/uploads/2016/10/2016-SGO-Genetics-Toolkit3.pdf

BREAST CANCER: Malignant tumor in breast tissue. P.107

http://www.jwatch.org/na44519/2017/07/06/asco-2017-report-breast-cancer?query=topic_breastcan&

jwd=000012066693&jspc=OBG
https://www.acog.org/-/media/Practice-Bulletins/
Committee-on-Practice-Bulletins----Gynecology/Public/
pb179.pdf?dmc=1&ts=20170710T0228314803
https://tools.bcsc-scc.org/BC5yearRisk/intro.htm
https://insights.ovid.com/crossref?
an=00006250-201709000-00035

BRONCHITIS: Inflammation of the bronchial passages.
P.268
https://www.ncbi.nlm.nih.gov/pubmed/23204254

BULEMIA: Eating disorder. Food consumption followed
by self-induced vomiting. P.55
https://www.ncbi.nlm.nih.gov/pmc/articles/
PMC2927890/

BUNDLE BRANCH BLOCK: Delay in the pathway of
electrical impulses to the left or right ventricle of the
heart, resulting in a delay of contraction of that ventricle.
http://www.acc.org/latest-in-cardiology/journal-scans
/2016/08/05/11/45/effect-of-the-antihypertensive-and-
lipid-lowering-treatment?w_nav=LC

CANCER: Malignant tumor (growth). The hallmark of
cancer is its ability to invade normal tissue. Cancer can
often metastasize, spreading to distant areas in the body.
It is likely to recur even though it has been removed or
destroyed at its initial (primary) site. P.93, 266.

http://www.cell.com/cell/fulltext/S0092-8674(18)3032-7

http://www.cell.com/pb-assets/consortium/pancancer-atlas/pancan/index.html

https://www.cancer.gov/about-cancer/treatment/types/targeted-therapies/targeted-therapies-fact-sheet

https://cancerstaging.org/About/news/Pages/-Cancer-Staging-Manual, -Eighth-Edition, -Just-Released-by-American-Joint-Committee-on-Cancer-(AJCC).aspx

http://www.jcso-ejournal.com/jcso/november_2016?pg=34#pg34

http://journal.frontiersin.org/article/10.3389/fimmu.2017.00374/full?utm_source=F-AAE&utm_medium=EMLF&utm_campaign=MRK_243180_20170411_arts

https://www.nature.com/articles/s41551-017-0067?WT.mc_id=EMI_NBME_1704_APRILISSUE_PORTFOLIO&spMailingID=53957850&spUserID=MTc3MDI4ODk5NQ

http://stm.sciencemag.org/content/9/400/eaan2966

http://science.sciencemag.org/content/early/2018/01/17/science.aar3247

CANCER MARKER: Substances produced by tumor cells or by other cells in response to a tumor. See: Tumor Specific Antigen (TSA). P.19, 119, 330, 331

https://www.nature.com/articles/s41551-017-0065?WT.mc_id=EMI_NBME_1704_APRILISSUE_PORTFOLIO&spMailingID=53957850&spUserID=MTc3MDI4ODk5NQS

CANNABIS: Plant from which cannabinoids are obtained. Tetrahydrocannabinol (THC) is the principal psychoactive compound. P.285
https://medicalmarijuana.procon.org/view.resource.php?resourceID=000141
https://www.ncbi.nlm.nih.gov/pubmed/16463612

CARBOHYDRATE: Simple and complex sugars that are the energy source for the body. Excess carbohydrate can be converted to fat for storage.
http://www.fao.org/docrep/w8079e/w8079e0h.htm

CARCINOGEN: Substance or radiation that predisposes to cancer
http://mdlinx.pdr.net/internal-medicine/news-article.cfm/6931990/?utm_source=in-house&utm_medium=message&utm_campaign=mh-im-nov16
https://en.wikipedia.org/wiki/Carcinogen

CARPAL TUNNEL SYNDROME : CTS: Restriction of the median nerve by the transverse carpal ligament at the wrist resulting in compression neuropathy.
https://www.ncbi.nlm.nih.gov/pmc/articles/PMC3314870/

CAR-T: Chimeric Antigen Receptor T-Cell therapy: T-cells genetically modified to enhance tumor destruction.
https://www.cancer.gov/about-cancer/treatment/research/car-t-cells

http://www.nejm.org/doi/full/10.1056/nejmoa1407222#t=
article

https://jhoonline.biomedcentral.com/articles/10.1186/
s13045-017-0423-1

www.empr.com/news/first-gene-therapy-antigen-receptor-t-
cell-acute-lymphoblastic-leukemia/article/685222/?DCMP=
EMC-MPR_DailyDose_cp_20170830&cpn=obgyn_all
https://jamanetwork.com/journals/jama/fullarticle
/2664338?utm_source=silverchair&utm_medium=email&
utm_campaign=article_alert-jama&utm_content=olf&
utm_term

The Promise and Challenges of CAR-T Gene Therapy |
Genetics and Genomics | JAMA | The JAMA Network

CAT SCAN: Computerized Axial Tomography. An
advanced, computerized imaging technique that very
quickly takes serial Xrays through the body in thin
"slices", so that very small abnormalities can be found.
With a helical (spiral) three dimensional CAT scan the
Xray tube revolves around the patient. A four dimensional CAT scan takes multiple images during phases of
the breathing cycle, particularly useful in cases of lung
tumors that have to be precisely localized and that move
with respiration. The fourth dimension is Time. P.35, 56,
90, 98, 99, 119, 142, 175, 244, 330, 331.
https://radiopaedia.org/articles/computed-tomography
http://www.jwatch.org/na43480/2017/03/16/

radiation-exposure-and-cancer-risk-low-dose-ct-lung-cancer?query=etoc_jwgenmed&jwd=000012066693&jspc=OBG

CATALYST: A substance that facilitates a chemical reaction without being changed by that reaction. P.34

CATARACT: Clouding, loss of transparency, of the lens of the eye. P.387, 388
http://www.webmd.com/eye-health/cataracts/extracapsular-surgery-for-cataracts

CAUTERY: (Electrocautery) Surgical destruction of tissue by direct current heating. **Electrosurgery** utilizes radio frequency (RF) alternating current to heat tissue. https://en.wikipedia.org/wiki/Electrosurgery

CELL: The basic living microscopic structure in the human body. Each cell is surrounded by a cell membrane. Cells generally have a center, the nucleus, which is itself surrounded by a membrane. The nucleus contains the chromosomes, on which rest the genes. https://en.wikipedia.org/wiki/Cell_(biology)

CEREBROVASCULAR ACCIDENT: See "Stroke" P.74

CERVICAL CANCER: Cancer of the uterine cervix. Most often caused by specific Types of sexually transmitted Human Papilloma Virus (**HPV**), which can also cause **carcinoma of the penis.** Largely preventable by **vaccines.**

https://www.ncbi.nlm.nih.gov/pubmed/12120445
https://www.cancer.gov/about-cancer/causes-prevention
/risk/infectious-agents/hpv-vaccine-fact-sheet
https://emedicine.medscape.com/article
/2006486-overview

CERVIX: The mouth, or neck, of the uterus, projecting
through the vaginal vault. Its opening is the cervical os.
P.124, 127

http://www.obgyn.net/gynecological-oncology/
identifying-squamous-cancer-colposcopy

CHECKPOINT: T-lymphocyte locus that can shut
off T-cell and suppress the immune response. (See
T-lymphocyte)

http://www.cgen.com/focus-areas/immuno-oncology/
immune-checkpoints

http://journal.frontiersin.org/article/10.3389/
fimmu.2017.00692/full?utm_source=F-AAE&utm_
medium=EMLF&utm_campaign=MRK_307979_35_
Immuno_20170622_arts_A

**CHECKPOINT INHIBITOR:(Immune Checkpoint
Inhibitor, ICI)** Drug that blocks a checkpoint, allowing
T-lymphocyte to respond to malignant cell. Ref: Pardoll,
Drew: Nature Reviews Cancer 12, 252-264 (April 2012)

http://blog.dana-farber.org/insight/2015/09/what-is-a-
checkpoint-inhibitor/

http://ascopubs.org/doi/full/10.1200/JCO.2017.74.6065

http://jamanetwork.com/journals/jama/fullarticle
/2653953?amp;utm_source=JAMAPublishAheadofPrint&
utm_campaign=08-09-2017
http://ard.bmj.com/content/76/10/1747

CHIMERA: A single organism composed of cells from
different zygotes. A **chimeric gene** combines portions of
different coding sequences to produce a new gene.

https://en.wikipedia.org/wiki/Chimeric_gene

CHIP: Clonal Hematopoiesis of Indeterminate Potential:
Acquired mutations in hematopoietic stem cells
that accumulate in bone marrow, associated with an
increased risk of heart attack and stroke
https://www.ncbi.nlm.nih.gov/pmc/articles/
PMC4961884/
 http://www.nejm.org/doi/full/10.1056/NEJMoa1701719

CHOLESTEROL: Normally occurring lipoproteins in
the body. If cholesterol levels, and levels of low density
lipoprotein (LDL) are too high, atherosclerosis can result.
P.64, 72, 77, 78, 79, 157, 211, 213
http://emedicine.medscape.com/article/121187-overview

CHOLESTEROL INHIBITOR: Drug that inhibits the
intestine from absorbing cholesterol. P.80
http://www.health.harvard.edu/blog/pcsk9-inhibitors-
a-major-advance-in-cholesterol-lowering-drug-ther-
apy-201503157801

CHORIONIC VILLI: Microscopic projections from the placenta in which fetal blood circulates. P.252
https://en.wikipedia.org/wiki/Chorionic_villus_ sampling

CHROMATIN: The protein (**histone**)/DNA complex in the cell nucleus that forms the chromosome.
https://en.wikipedia.org/wiki/Chromatin
http://www.nature.com/news/plot-a-course-through-the-genome-1.22553?WT.ec_id=NATURE-20170907&spMailingID=54864391&spUserID=MjA1NjIyNjc4OAS2&spJobID=1244089361&spReportId=MTI0NDA4OTM2MQS2

CHROMOSOME: An elongated, stringlike structure in the nucleus of the cell that carries the genes. There are forty six chromosomes in each cell, arranged in twenty three pairs. One of each pair is originally derived from the mother, and one from the father. P.18, 22, 23, 29, 32, 34, 41, 48
https://www.genome.gov/26524120/chromosomes-fact-sheet/

CILIA: Tiny hairlike projections on cells. P.36, 356.

CIRCADIAN RHYTHM: Biologic process that exhibits endogenous circadian (24 hour, diurnal) cycle. Can be influenced by external factors.
https://www.ncbi.nlm.nih.gov/pmc/articles/ PMC4353305/
https://en.wikipedia.org/wiki/Circadian_rhythm

CIRRHOSIS: Chronic degeneration of liver cells accompanied by fibrous scarring of the liver. P.290
https://www.niddk.nih.gov/health-information/health-topics/liver-disease/cirrhosis/Pages/facts.aspx

CLITORIS: The erectile organ above the urethral orifice at the entrance to the vagina. P.124
https://www.ncbi.nlm.nih.gov/pubmed/23169570

CLONE: An exact genetic copy. An identical twin is a clone because the fertilized egg splits in two. A fraternal twin is not a clone because two different eggs, fertilized by two different sperm develop in the uterus at the same time. P.43, 46
https://www.genome.gov/25020028/cloning-fact-sheet/
http://www.cell.com/cell/fulltext/S0092-8674(18)30057-6

COCHLEAR IMPLANT: Medical device that replaces the function of the inner ear, sends signals to the brain via the auditory nerve. P.269
https://www.nidcd.nih.gov/health/cochlear-implants

COGNITION: Conscious mental activities of thinking, learning, understanding and remembering. P.175, 203
https://www.sciencedaily.com/releases/2016/09/160909095045.htm
http://psychcentral.com/lib/in-depth-cognitive-behavioral-therapy/
https://www.mdlinx.com/family-medicine/

medical-news-article/2016/12/13/coffee-chlorogenic-
acid-vascular-phenolics-flow-mediated-dilatation-fmd-
/6965864/?category=last-month&page_id=1
http://journal.frontiersin.org/article/10.3389/
fimmu.2017.01101/full?utm_source=F-AAE&utm_
medium=EMLF&utm_campaign=MRK_398354_35_
Immuno_20170921_arts_A

COGNITIVE IMPAIRMENT: Mild Cognitive
Impairment (**MCI**) is a dysfunction of conscious mental
activities with minimal impairment of the instrumental
activities of daily life (IADL). In Amnestic MCI memory
dysfunction predominates. There can be progression to
Dementia. The Care of the Older Person: "Doctor, my
wife is getting forgetful": Serge Gauthier ; Management
of older patients in the Emergency Department: Cyrille
Launay ; Assessment of decision-making capacity:
Catherine Ferrier.
http://n.neurology.org/content/90/3/126
http://n.neurology.org/content/90/13/e1158

https://academic.oup.com/brain/
article/141/3/877/4818093

COLON, COLORECTAL CANCER: Cancer of the large
intestine and rectum. Detectable at precancerous and
early stage by colonoscopy and biopsy. Cancer markers
can be used in screening.
https://www.ncbi.nlm.nih.gov/pubmed/26151224

https://emedicine.medscape.com/article/1948929-overview

https://cancerstaging.org/references-tools/quickreferences/Documents/ColonMedium.pdf

https://www.cancer.org/cancer/colon-rectal-cancer/detection-diagnosis-staging/how-diagnosed.html

https://gi.org/guideline/colorectal-cancer-screening-recommendations-for-physicians-and-patients-from-the-us-multi-society-task-force-on-colorectal-cancer/

COLONOSCOPY: Direct inspection of the entire large intestine with a flexible fiberoptic instrument called a colonoscope. P.118

http://www.asge.org/assets/0/71328/9cf71f1d-ef18-4a34-9259-31f487a6213c.pdf

COLOR FLOW DOPPLER: Ultrasound with color coding of blood flow velocity and direction. Doppler effect refers to the measurable difference in sound as it moves away. P.141

https://123sonography.com/content/1821-principles-color-doppler

COMA: Deep, unarousable unconsciousness
https://www.medicinenet.com/script/main/art.asp?articlekey=2803

https://www.ncbi.nlm.nih.gov/pubmed/19001840

CONCUSSION: Traumatic injury to the brain.
https://www.cdc.gov/headsup/basics/concussion_wha-
tis.html
https://www.cdc.gov/traumaticbraininjury/severe.html
https://www.fda.gov/NewsEvents/Newsroom/
PressAnnouncements/ucm596531.htm

CORD BLOOD: Fetal blood in the umbilical cord. Can
be banked in order to retrieve stem cells . P.42
http://www.acog.org/Resources-And-Publications
/Committee-Opinions/Committee-on-Genetics/
Umbilical-Cord-Blood-Banking

COX-1 INHIBITOR: Drugs including aspirin, ibuprofen,
and Naprosyn are both COX-1 and COX-2 inhibitors,
inhibiting cyclooxygenase-I as well as cyclooxygenase 2.
P.67, 115, 165
http://www.ncbi.nlm.nih.gov/pubmed/11566042

COX-2 INHIBITOR: Non-steroidal anti-inflammatory
drugs (NSAID's). These drugs target cyclooxygenase-2
(COX-2) enzyme that encourages prostaglandin production, leading to inflammation and pain.   P.115, 163, 165
http://journal.frontiersin.org/article/10.3389/
fimmu.2016.00375/full?utm_source=newsletter&utm_
medium=email&utm_campaign=Immunology-w40-2016

C-REACTIVE PROTEIN: CRP. Plasma protein with
increased concentration in the presence of inflammatory

disorders. The Care of the Older Person: Could My
Patient be Malnourished ?: Jose Morais.   P.205
https://en.wikipedia.org/wiki/C-reactive_protein
https://www.ncbi.nlm.nih.gov/pubmed/11532280
http://www.mdedge.com/oncologypractice/article
/147564/immuno-oncology/crp-may-predict-survival-
after-immunotherapy-lung?channel=240&utm_source=
News_OP_sf-lung

CRISP R: Clustered **R**egularly **I**nterspaced **S**hort
Palindromic **R**epeats. Segments of **prokaryotic** DNA
containing repetitions of base sequences, followed by
segments of spacer DNA. Used in **genome editing**.
CRISPR-Cas9 : Complex of RNA and protein (nucleases):
Recognizes sequence of bases in target gene. Cas9 (an
enzyme) unwinds double helix. CRISPR RNA sequence
binds to target. Cas9 cuts both strands of target DNA.
In a modification, DNA sequences are not cut: the Cas9
enzyme carries a molecular switch that turns on target
genes.
http://www.ncbi.nlm.nih.gov/pmc/articles/PMC4786927/
http://link.springer.com/article/10.1186/s12977-016-0270-
0?view=classic
http://www.bloomberg.com/features/2016-how-crispr-
will-change-the-world/
http://jamanetwork.com/journals/jama/article-abstract
/2600454
https://en.wikipedia.org/wiki/CRISPR

http://journal.frontiersin.org/article/10.3389/
fimmu.2016.00375/full?utm_source=newsletter&utm_
medium=email&utm_campaign=Immunology-w40-2016
https://www.technologyreview.com/s/608350/first-
human-embryos-edited-in-us/
http://jamanetwork.com/journals/jama/fullar-
ticle/2646800?utm_medium=alert&utm_source=
JAMAPublishAheadofPrint&utm_campaign=10-08-2017
https://www.nature.com/news/crispr-hacks-enable-
pinpoint-repairs-to-genome-1.22884?WT.ec_id=
NATURE-20171026&spMailingID=55217903&spUserID=
MjA1
https://www.ncbi.nlm.nih.gov/pubmed/27052831
http://www.cell.com/cell/fulltext/S0092-8674(17)31247-3

https://www.google.com/url?hl=en&q=http://links.
information.nature.com/ctt?kn%3D44%26ms%3D-
NTYxMDY0ODYS1%26r%3DMjk1NTYwNTAxN-
zA4S0%26b%3D0%26j%

CRYOSURGERY: Surgical destruction of tissue by freez-
ing.
http://emedicine.medscape.com/article/1125851-overview

CUL DE SAC: Rectouterine peritoneal pouch between
the posterior wall of the uterus and the rectum. P.125, 248
https://en.wikipedia.org/wiki/Recto-uterine_pouch

CYBERNETICS: Control and communication with living tissue, as with a chip implanted in a muscle. P.269
http://www.asc-cybernetics.org/foundations/definitions.htm

CYST: A fluid-filled growth (tumor). May be benign or malignant.
https://www.ncbi.nlm.nih.gov/pubmed/21845969
http://www.pathologyoutlines.com/topic/ovarytumor-whoclassif.html

CYSTOCELE: Bulge of the urinary bladder into the anterior wall of the vagina. P.234
https://www.niddk.nih.gov/health-information/health-topics/urologic-disease/cystocele/Pages/facts.aspx

CYSTOSCOPE: Operating telescope used to visualize the interior of the urinary bladder and the ureteral orifices. P. 237, 238. See : The Care of the Older Person: Incontinence in Older Adults : Samer Shamout, Lysanne Campeau.
https://www.ncbi.nlm.nih.gov/pmc/articles/PMC4457046/
https://en.wikipedia.org/wiki/Cystoscopy

CYTOKINE: Factor released by a cell that has an effect on other cells. P.249
http://www.ncbi.nlm.nih.gov/pmc/articles/PMC2785020/

http://journal.frontiersin.org/article/10.3389/
fimmu.2017.00930/full?utm_source=F-AAE&utm_
medium=EMLF&utm_campaign=MRK_352999_35_
Immuno_20170808_arts_A
https://www.frontiersin.org/articles/10.3389/
fimmu.2018.00422/full?utm_source=F-AAE&utm_
medium=EMLF&utm_campaign=MRK_571163_35_I

https://www.frontiersin.org/articles/10.3389/
fimmu.2018.00586/full?utm_source=F-AAE&utm_medi-
um=EMLF&utm_campaign=MRK_608868_35_I

CYTOPLASM: The contents of a cell outside the nucleus.
https://en.wikipedia.org/wiki/Cytoplasm

DEEP LEARNING: Deep neural network model.
Machine learning technique analyzing large amounts of
data, enabling prediction of outcomes (prognosis) when
new data is presented. May be used to predict cardiovascular disease risk by observation of the eye retina.
https://arxiv.org/abs/1708.09843
https://en.wikipedia.org/wiki/Deep_learning

DELIRIUM: Confusional state with altered attention
and awareness. See: The Care of the Older Person: How
to Diagnose and Manage Delirium: Haibin Yin.
https://www.ncbi.nlm.nih.gov/pubmed/25300023
https://www.uptodate.com/contents/
diagnosis-of-delirium-and-confusional-states

DELIVERY: The birth of the baby as it exits the birth canal. P.232

DEMENTIA: Loss of cognitive functioning. P.203, 298. Frontotemporal Dementia refers to a heterogenous group of conditions. See: The Care of the Older Person: Dementia: "Doctor, My Wife is Getting Forgetful": Serge Gauthier; How do I protect my patient? Randy S. Perskin http://www.ncbi.nlm.nih.gov/pmc/articles/PMC2211335/ http://www.bmj.com/content/347/bmj.f4827 https://www.jwatch.org/na45523/2017/12/05/healthy-life-healthy-brain-lifestyle-factors-and-dementia?query= etoc_jwneuro&jwd=000012066693&jspc=OBG http://n.neurology.org/content/90/3/126 http://geropsychiatriceducation.vch.ca/docs/edu-down-loads/depression/cornell_scale_depression.pdf https://www.bmj.com/content/361/bmj.k1315

DEMOGRAPHY: The study of groups of people and their environment. http://www.pewresearch.org/fact-tank/2016/03/31/10-demographic-trends-that-are-shaping-the-u-s-and-the-world/

DEPRESSION: Depressive disorder marked by prolonged sadness, mood alteration, often with feelings of loss, anger and frustration. See: The Care of the Older Person: An Overview of Late-Life Depression: Artin Mahdanian, Silvia Monti De Flores. P.214, 218, 332

http://www.ncbi.nlm.nih.gov/pmc/articles/PMC2922383/
http://geropsychiatriceducation.vch.ca/docs/edu-down-
loads/depression/cornell_scale_depression.pdf

DERMABRASION: Surgical procedure to remove skin
imperfections by abrading the skin surface. P.393
http://emedicine.medscape.com/article
/1297069-treatment

DETRUSOR MUSCLE: Muscular coat of the urinary
bladder. P.237. See: The Care of the Older Person :
Incontinence In Older Adults : Samer Shamout, Lysanne
Campeau
http://emedicine.medscape.com/article/1949017-overview

DHEA: Dehydroepiandrosterone. Androgenic steroid
hormone secreted largely by adrenal cortex. P.158, 205,
244, 391
https://en.wikipedia.org/wiki/Dehydroepiandrosterone

DIABETES MELLITUS: Chronic disease characterized
by abnormally high blood glucose levels. P.151, 265, 266,
270, 282, 295, 327, 328. See: The Care of the Older Person:
Could My Patient Be Malnourished ? : Jose Morais
; Frailty : Sathya Karunananthan, Howard Bergman
; Polypharmacy And Deprescribing In The Elderly :
Louise Mallet
http://www.merckmanuals.com/profes-
sional/endocrine-and-metabolic-disorders/

diabetes-mellitus-and-disorders-of-carbohydrate-metab-olism/diabetes-mellitus-dm

DIET: Food intake. P.9 See: The Care of the Older Person : Could My Patient Be Malnourished ? : Jose Morais. http://www.pubfacts.com/detail/27465379/Relation-between-mealtime-distribution-of-protein-intake-and-lean-mass-loss-in-free-living-older-adu http://jamanetwork.com/journals/jama/fullarticle /2636710

DIURETIC: Drug that causes increased passage of fluid by the kidneys. P.74. See: The Care of the Older Person : Polypharmacy And Deprescribing In The Elderly : Louise Mallet ; Incontinence In Older Adults: Samer Shamout , Louise Campeau http://emedicine.medscape.com/article /2145340-overview

DNA: Deoxyribonucleic acid. DNA makes up the chro-mosomes that carry the genes. DNA is arranged in a distinctive double helix , three dimensional pattern. It resembles a tight spiral staircase, with rungs (steps) each of which holds two (out of four) nucleic acid bases, called **base pairs.** P.22, 33, 34, 120, 121 https://www.genome.gov/25520880/deoxyribonucleic-acid-dna-fact-sheet/

DNA MICROARRAY: DNA Biochip. Collection of microscopic DNA spots on a surface. Used to measure gene expression patterns.
https://www.genome.gov/10000533/dna-microarray-technology/

DNA MISMATCH REPAIR: During DNA replication, erroneous insertion, deletion and misincorporation of bases can occur in the daughter DNA strand. Such errors can also occur during DNA recombination. DNA Mismatch Repair involves the recognition and correction of these abnormalities.
https://en.wikipedia.org/wiki/DNA_mismatch_repair
https://jamanetwork.com/journals/jamasurgery/article-abstract/2647248?utm_medium=alert&utm_source=JAMA+SurgLatestIssue&utm_campaign=15-11-2017
https://www.nature.com/scitable/topicpage/dna-is-constantly-changing-through-the-process-6524876

DNA PROBE: A highly specific test to detect the DNA of an individual, or a virus. It is used to detect the human papilloma virus (HPV) that is the usual causative organism of cancer of the cervix. The test is used in the criminal investigation of rape, and in identification. An individual male can be identified by the distinctive DNA in his sperm. P.XII, 39, 130, 331
http://www.nature.com/subjects/dna-probesv

DOPAMINE: A neurotransmitter. P.181
http://www.dictionary.com/browse/dopamine

DUODENUM: First part of the small intestine after the stomach. P.358
http://emedicine.medscape.com/article
/1948951-overview

DYSKINESIA: Abnormality of voluntary movement. P.179, 180
https://en.wikipedia.org/wiki/Dyskinesia

DYSMENORRHEA: Pain with menses. P.190
https://academic.oup.com/epirev/article/36/1/104/566554

DYSPAREUNIA: Painful intercourse. P.224
https://www.ncbi.nlm.nih.gov/pmc/articles/
PMC2671314/

DYSPLASIA: An abnormal, benign, microscopic cell change that can be a precursor of cancer. P.149
http://www.cancer.gov/publications/dictionaries/cancer-terms?cdrid=45675

ECTOPIC PREGNANCY: Pregnancy outside of the normal location in the uterus. Usually in a fallopian tube. P. 126
https://academic.oup.com/humupd/article/20/2/250
/663951

EDEMA: Swelling by accumulation of fluid in tissues. P.302. See: The Care of the Older Person : Could My

Patient Be Malnourished ? : Jose Morais
http://www.ncbi.nlm.nih.gov/books/NBK53445/

ELDER ABUSE: The intentional or neglectful causing
of harm to an aging person See: The Care of the Older
Person: Elder Abuse: Mark J. Yaffe
https://online.epocrates.com/diseases/69735/Elder-abuse
/Differential-Diagnosis

ELECTROCARDIOGRAM: Noninvasive test that measures the electrical activity of the heart. P.69, 331
https://www.ncbi.nlm.nih.gov/pmc/articles/PMC1614214/

EMBOLIZATION: Therapeutic introduction of a
substance into a blood vessel to occlude it. P.147.
Transcatheter Arterial Chemoembolization (TACE)
combines the introduction of therapeutic substances into
a tumor in conjunction with occlusion of the blood vessels of the tumor.
http://www.hopkinsmedicine.org/liver_tumor_center/
treatments/intraarterial_therapies/tace.html

EMBOLUS: Detached thrombus (blood clot) that travels
through blood vessels to another site. P.89, 109, 179, 204
http://emedicine.medscape.com/article/300901-overview
http://emedicine.medscape.com/article
/1916852-overview

EMBRYO: The developing baby in the uterus during the
fourth to eighth weeks of development, to the end of the

second month, by which time all major features of the body are recognizable. All the main organ systems in the body have been laid down by the end of the second month. P.VIII, 44, 47
https://embryology.med.unsw.edu.au/embryology/index.php/Ultrasound

EMOTION: Affective state of consciousness. Feeling. P.332
https://www.ncbi.nlm.nih.gov/pmc/articles/PMC3950961/

ENDOCRINE GLANDS: Glands that secrete (produce) hormones, including the pituitary gland at the base of the brain, the thyroid gland, the adrenal glands , the ovaries, and the testes.
https://en.wikipedia.org/wiki/Endocrine_gland

ENDOCYTOSIS: Active transport of molecules into the cell in an energy using process
https://www.ncbi.nlm.nih.gov/books/NBK9831/

ENDOMETRIAL BIOPSY: Surgical sampling of the uterine lining. P.135, 194, 245
https://academic.oup.com/humupd/article/23/2/232/2632344

ENDOMETRIAL CANCER: Cancer of the lining of the uterus.
https://www.ncbi.nlm.nih.gov/pmc/articles/PMC5288678/

ENDOMETRIAL HYPERPLASIA: Benign over- growth condition of the lining of the uterus with crowding of glands. **ATYPICAL (ADENOMATOUS) HYPERPLASIA** of the endometrium is considered to be premalignant.
https://pdfs.semanticscholar.org/3b81/8cfedf864fca863 c378a8028f91e0280b299.pdf

ENDOMETRIOSIS: Abnormal deposition of endome- trium outside the uterus. P.248
http://www.gponline.com/clinical-review-endometriosis /womens-health/endometriosis-fibroids/article/1150448

ENDOMETRIUM: The lining of the uterus. P.135

ENDORPHINS: Hormones that affect receptors in the brain. May reduce pain by binding to opioid receptors. P.217
http://www.ncbi.nlm.nih.gov/pmc/articles/PMC3104618 /

ENDOTHELIN I: A vasoconstrictor. P.290
http://www.ncbi.nlm.nih.gov/pmc/articles/PMC3005421 /

ENTEROCELE: True hernia of small bowel covered by peritoneum bulging into the vaginal vault. P.234, 240

ENZYME: An organic catalyst. Enzymes facilitate chem- ical reactions within the human body. P.34, 69 https://www.mcat.me/review/bb/enzyme-structure-and-function/

EPF: Early Pregnancy Factor. Pregnancy-specific protein that is present in pregnant woman's serum 48 hours after fertilization. P. 253
http://www.ncbi.nlm.nih.gov/pubmed/9196793

EPIDEMIC: Increase in the number of cases of a disease in a population.
https://www.cdc.gov/ophss/csels/dsepd/ss1978/lesson1/section11.html
https://www.hhs.gov/opioids/about-the-epidemic/index.html

EPIDIDYMIS: Duct behind the testis that carries sperm to the vas deferens. P.247
http://emedicine.medscape.com/article/1949259-overview

EPIGENOME: Chemical modifications to DNA and DNA-associated proteins in the cell which alter gene expression. Epigenetic changes can drive aging. Much of the epigenome is reset when the genome is passed to offspring.
https://www.genome.gov/27532724/
http://www.nature.com/news/an-epigenetics-gold-rush-new-controls-for-gene-expression-1.21513?WT.ec_id=

NATURE-20170223&spMailingID=53480287&spUserID=
MjA1NjIyNjc4OA

EPITHELIUM: A microscopic cellular covering of surfaces, including skin and mucous membranes.
http://anatomyandphysiologyi.com/epithelial-tissue/

EPITOPE: Antigenic determinant. The part of the antigen molecule that is recognized by the antibody, and to
which the antibody attaches.
https://www.britannica.com/science/epitope

ERECTILE DYSFUNCTION: ED. Difficulty with achiev-
ing or maintaining penile erection. P.223
http://www.bmj.com/content/348/bmj.g129

ERYTHROPOIETIN: Stimulates the formation of red blood
cells. Produced by recombinant DNA technology. P.40
https://en.wikipedia.org/wiki/Erythropoietin

ESTRADIOL: A form of estrogen produced in the ovaries.
https://pubchem.ncbi.nlm.nih.gov/compound/estradiol

ESTROGEN: Female sex hormones, mainly made in the
ovary. P.69, 146, 188, 201, 203, 237, 244, 250, 253, 293, 394
https://en.wikipedia.org/wiki/Estrogen
http://journal.frontiersin.org/article/10.3389/
fimmu.2017.00108/full?utm_source=newsletter&utm_
medium=email&utm_campaign=Immunology-w7-2017

ESTROGEN REPLACEMENT THERAPY: ERT. Treatment of menopausal symptoms, usually in conjunction with progesterone. P.137, 179
http://emedicine.medscape.com/article/276104-overview

EUKARYOTE: Any organism whose cells contain a nucleus which contains DNA within chromosomes.
http://www.dictionary.com/browse/eukaryote

EXERCISE (AEROBIC): Generally refers to sustained physical activity designed to promote oxygen utilization. The Care of the Older Person: Why Does My Patient Have Gait and Balance Disorders ?: Olivier Beauchet. P.74, 311
http://cardiology.jamanetwork.com/article.aspx?
articleid=2530563

FABRY'S DISEASE: Alpha-galactosidase-A deficiency: enzyme utilized in lipid metabolism. Rare X-linked lysosomal storage disease. P. 27
http://www.ninds.nih.gov/disorders/fabrys/fabrys.htm

FALLOPIAN TUBE: The fine tubular structure arising from each side of the uterus near the fundus, ending in fingerlike projections called fimbria that are close to each ovary, essentially forming the "pickup" mechanism for the egg released at ovulation. P.125, 246, 249, 269

FERTILITY: The ability to conceive children. P.243
http://emedicine.medscape.com/article/274143-overview

FERTILIZATION: The fusion of the ovum (oocyte, egg) and the spermatozoon (sperm). P. 194, 247
https://en.wikipedia.org/wiki/Human_fertilization

FETUS: The baby developing in the uterus is known as the fetus from the beginning of the third month until the baby is born. The fetal period is the longest period of intrauterine life. P.259
http://www.nature.com/news/secrets-of-life-in-a-spoon-ful-of-blood-1.21430?WT.ec_id=NATURE-20170209&spMailingID=53380605&spUserID=MjA1NjIyNjc4OAS2&spJobID=1101425398&spReportId=MTEwMTQyNTM5OAS2

FHIT GENE: Fragile histidine triad. Aberrant transcripts from this gene are found in some cancers, notably esophageal, stomach and colon cancer. P.107
http://www.ncbi.nlm.nih.gov/gene/2272

FIBEROPTICS: Light images sent through fine fibers of glass or plastic. P.3, 194
http://www.laserfocusworld.com/articles/2011/01/medical-applications-of-fiber-optics-optical-fiber-sees-growth-as-medical-sensors.html

FIBRIN: In blood clotting, thrombin causes fibrinogen to polymerize, forming fibrin. Polymerized fibrin and platelets form a hemostatic plug , or clot, P.255
https://www.britannica.com/science/fibrin

FIBROID: A benign solid tumor of the uterus. P. 145

FIBROMA: A benign solid tumor that can occur in the breast or ovary.

FISTULA: An abnormal passage from one body cavity to another, or out to the body surface. P.232

FOLLICLE (OVARIAN): The fluid-filled structure surrounding the developing egg (ovum)in the ovary. P.245
http://www.embryology.ch/anglais/cgametogen/oogenese02.html

FRAILTY SYNDROME: Weakness, slowness, minimal physical activity, exhaustion and low energy, weight loss. See: The Care of the Older Person: Frailty: Sathya Karunananthan, Howard Bergman
https://jamanetwork.com/journals/jamasurgery/article-abstract/2656841
http://www.ncbi.nlm.nih.gov/pubmed/17634320
http://annals.org/aim/article-abstract/2668215/effect-physical-activity-frailty-secondary-analysis-randomized-controlled-trial

FREE RADICAL: Short lived uncharged molecule. P.284
http://www.ncbi.nlm.nih.gov/pmc/articles/PMC3249911/

FSH: Follicle stimulating hormone. P.186, 188, 192, 244, 250
http://www.ncbi.nlm.nih.gov/pubmed/9741710

GABA: Gamma-aminobutyric acid. A neurotransmitter. P. 220

http://www.webmd.com/vitamins-supplements/ingre-dientmono-464-gaba%20gamma-aminobutyric%20acid.aspx?activeingredientid=464&

GALACTOGRAPHY: Mammography with injection of contrast to image milk ducts. P.112

GAMETE: A germ (sex) cell: the female ovum, or the male spermatozoon. https://www.khanacademy.org/science/biology/cellular-molecular-biology/meiosis/a/phases-of-meiosis

GENE: The determinant of human characteristics and behavior from a cellular level on upwards. Each gene is a section on a DNA molecule and usually resides at a specific point (locus) on a chromosome. Each gene has a counterpart on the other chromosome that makes up the pair. The genes elaborate proteins. P.18, 22, 34, 180 http://www.ncbi.nlm.nih.gov/genbank/

GENE EDITING (Genome Editing): A form of **Genetic Engineering.** Insertion, deletion or replacement of DNA at a specific site on the genome using engineered nucle-ases ("molecular scissors") See **CRISP R** https://www.technologyreview.com/s/608350/first-human-embryos-edited-in-us/ https://www.horizondiscovery.com/gene-editing

http://jamanetwork.com/journals/jama/fullar-
ticle/2646800?utm_medium=alert&utm_source=
JAMAPublishAheadofPrint&utm_campaign=10-08-2017

GENE EXPRESSION PROFILING: Measurement of
activity (expression) of thousands of genes, giving a pic-
ture of cellular functioning. In breast cancer for example,
identifies distinct molecular entities associated with differential prognoses and response to cytotoxic drugs.
http://www.ncbi.nlm.nih.gov/pubmed/11823860
http://www.mdedge.com/oncologypractice/clinical-
edge/summary/breast-cancer/optimizing-gene-expres-
sion-profiling-early-bc?utm_source=ClinEdge_OP_
cedge_110816&utm_medium=email&utm_content=
Gene%20Profiling%20in%20Early%20BC%20|%20CTC%20
Clusters%20and%20MBC%20|%20Impact%20of%20
Chemo%20Events%20|%20&%20More%20ClinicalEdge

GENE SILENCING: Regulation of gene expression. P.284
http://www.ncbi.nlm.nih.gov/probe/docs/applsilencing/

GENE THERAPY: Treating a disorder by inserting a
gene into cells. P.VIII, 27, 37, 71, 106, 151
http://www.ama-assn.org/ama/pub/physician-resources
/medical-science/genetics-molecular-medicine/current-
topics/gene-therapy.page?

https://www.frontiersin.org/arti-
cles/10.3389/fimmu.2018.00554/

full?utm_source=F-AAE&utm_medium=EMLF&utm_
campaign=MRK_589856_35_Immuno_20180403_arts_A

GENETIC ENGINEERING: Manipulating the genome.
P.292

http://www.fda.gov/AnimalVeterinary/
DevelopmentApprovalProcess/GeneticEngineering/
https://www.frontiersin.org/articles/10.3389/
fimmu.2018.00153/full?utm_source=F-AAE&utm_
medium=EMLF&utm_campaign=MRK_536191_35

GENOME: The complete DNA sequence. The human
genome project deciphered the complete DNA sequence
of humans. P.22, 32, 33, 35, 38

http://www.ncbi.nlm.nih.gov/projects/genome/guide/
human/

NEXT-GENERATION SEQUENCING: Technologies
that sample multiple DNA sequences in parallel.
https://www.cancer.gov/publications/dictionaries/genet-
ics-dictionary/def/next-generation-sequencing

GENOTYPE: The individual genes of each person. P.
XV, 22, 26, 173. **SNP genotyping** refers to variations in
Single Nucleotide Polymorphisms between individuals.
https://www.niehs.nih.gov/news/assets/docs_p_z/snp_
genotyping_508.pdf
http://www.nature.com/tpj/journal/v3/n2/full/6500167
a.html

GERD: Gastroesophageal Reflux Disease.
https://gi.org/guideline/diagnosis-and-managemen-of-
gastroesophageal-reflux-disease/

GERIATRICS: Medical specialty that focuses on health
care , diseases, and issues of elderly people, and the aging
process. See: The Care of the Older Person: Introduction:
Jose Morais
http://www.merckmanuals.com/professional/geriatrics/
provision-of-care-to-the-elderly/overview-of-geriatric-care
http://bulletin.facs.org/2016/12/improving-quality-in-
geriatric-surgery-a-blueprint-from-the-american-college-
of-surgeons/

GERONTOLOGY: The multidisciplinary study of aging
and its issues in all its aspects
http://biomedgerontology.oxfordjournals.org/content/59
/1/M24.full

GEROPROTECTOR: Drug that targets the fundamental
mechanisms of aging
https://www.nature.com/articles/d41586-018-01668-0?
utm_source=briefing-dy&utm_medium=email&
amp;utm_campaign=20180215

GLAND: Organ that synthesizes and secretes a substance required by the body.
http://www.histology.leeds.ac.uk/glandular/exocr_
endocr_properties.php

GLAUCOMA: Condition that causes optic nerve damage and vision loss, often by an increase in intraocular pressure. P.388

https://www.ncbi.nlm.nih.gov/pubmed/24825645vg

GLOBULINS: Include **alpha globulins,** beta **globulin,** and **gamma globulin, including (Ig)A, (Ig)G : immunoglobulin G , (Ig)M, (Ig)E and (Ig)D** synthesized by B lymphocytes, important in the immune response. Identified by **serum protein electrophoresis,** which separates the proteins.

https://www.aafp.org/afp/2005/0101/p105.html

https://www.ncbi.nlm.nih.gov/pmc/articles/PMC2715434/

https://www.reference.com/science/gamma-globulin-2944770f90b33e6c?aq=Gamma+Globulins&qo=cdpArticles

GLOBUS PALLIDUS: A subcortical structure in the brain. Part of the basal ganglia. P.181 .

http://webspace.ship.edu/cgboer/basalganglia.html

GLOMERULONEPHRITIS: Lesions of kidney glomeruli (capillary networks that filter blood) resulting from deposition or formation of immune complexes. In the acute phase, hematuria (blood in the urine), proteinuria (protein in the urine), and red blood cell casts in the urine are seen.

http://emedicine.medscape.com/article/239278-over-view#a4

http://www.sci.utah.edu/~macleod/bioen/be6000/prev-notes/L18-kidney.pdf

GOITER: Enlargement of the thyroid gland. P.299
http://www.uptodate.com/contents/
clinical-presentation-and-evaluation-of-goiter-in-adults

GNRH: Gonadotropin releasing hormone from the hypothalamus. P.145, 186, 250
http://emedicine.medscape.com/article/255152-overview

GRAFT: Healthy tissue taken from one part of the body to replace diseased or damaged tissue in another part. P.271

GRANULOSA CELL: A cell in the lining of an ovarian follicle. Granulosa cells manufacture estrogen, and to a lesser extent androgens and progestins. Conversion of androgens to estrogen takes place in granulosa cells. P.187, 192
https://embryology.med.unsw.edu.au/embryology/index.php/Granulosa_cell

GREENHOUSE GASES: Include carbon dioxide, sulfur dioxide, nitrous oxide, methane. P.5
https://www.epa.gov/ghgemissions/
overview-greenhouse-gases

GROWTH HORMONE: Somatotropin. Secreted by the pituitary gland. P.210

http://www.ncbi.nlm.nih.gov/pubmed/20020365

HCG: Human chorionic gonadotropin. Produced by the placenta. P.253

http://www.fda.gov/Drugs/ResourcesForYou
/Consumers/BuyingUsingMedicineSafely/
MedicationHealthFraud/ucm281834.htm

HEART FAILURE: Congestive heart failure. Heart muscle contraction not sufficiently strong to properly circulate blood. Fluid accumulates.

http://heartfailure.onlinejacc.org/article.aspx?
articleid=1568320

HEMORRHAGE: Excessive bleeding. P.264

HER-2 GENE: Human Epidermal Growth Factor Receptor-2. Linked to breast cancer. P.94

http://www.cancer.gov/research/progress/discovery/
HER2

HEREDITY: Parent to child transmission of traits, by inheritance of genes.

https://ghr.nlm.nih.gov/primer/inheritance/
inheritancepatterns

HERNIA: Intraabdominal contents enclosed by peritoneum bulging into a weakened wall. P.234

HIGH DENSITY LIPOPROTEIN: HDL. Complex of lipids and proteins that transports cholesterol in the blood to the liver. P.78, 154, 156, 159, 201
http://www.ncbi.nlm.nih.gov/pmc/articles/PMC3787738/
https://www.jwatch.org/na45882/2018/01/17/continuing-enigma-hdl?query=topic_lipid&jwd=000012066693&jspc=OBG

HIPPOCAMPUS: Area of the brain involved with spatial memory which is important in navigation, and episodic memory (remembering autobiographical events). Located in the medial temporal lobe of the brain. Includes a gray matter ridge on the floor of each lateral ventricle.
https://en.wikipedia.org/wiki/Hippocampus
https://www.nature.com/nature/journal/vaop/ncurrent/full/nature22067.html
https://en.wikipedia.org/wiki/Episodic_memory

HIRSUTISM: Excess hair growth. P.225, 250, 392
http://emedicine.medscape.com/article/121038-overview

HISTOCOMPATIBILITY: Antigenic similarities between tissue donor and recipient so that a transplant is not rejected. P.253
https://www.hindawi.com/journals/jtrans/2012/842141/

HMO: Health maintenance organization. Essentially a health insurance plan. P.56, 99, 362

HOLOGRAPHY: The scattered light from an object is captured, then illuminated by a beam. Multiple two dimensional pictures are assembled into a three dimensional display.
http://holocenter.org/what-is-holography

HOMOCYSTEINE: Amino acid derived from the dietary amino acid methionine. Homologue of the amino acid cysteine. P.85, 298
http://www.ncbi.nlm.nih.gov/pmc/articles/PMC4146172/

HOMOGRAFT: Transplanted tissue from another human individual. P. 251
http://bja.oxfordjournals.org/content/108/suppl_1/i29.full

HORMONE: A substance formed in an endocrine gland and carried by the blood stream to other organs which it affects. Such organs are called end organs. For example, follicle stimulating hormone and luteinizing hormone from the pituitary gland act on the ovary, controlling ovarian secretion of estrogen and progesterone. Estrogen and progesterone act on the endometrium lining the uterus.
http://biology.freeoda.com/chemical_composition_of_the_hormones.htm
http://www.news-medical.net/health/Hormone-Interactions-with-Receptors.aspx

HORMONE REPLACEMENT THERAPY: HRT. Treatment of menopausal symptoms with estrogen and

progesterone. P. 84, 184, 189, 196, 199, 209, 224, 327
http://press.endocrine.org/doi/abs/10.1210/jc.2015-2236

HOT FLASHES: Sudden onset of a feeling of heat and flushing of short duration. P.188, 202, 217, 250
http://theoncologist.alphamedpress.org/content/16/11
/1658.long

HUMAN CONNECTOME PROJECT: Mapping the human brain connectivity
http://www.humanconnectomeproject.org/

HYALURONIC ACID: An anionic nonsulfated glycosaminoglycan. Component of skin. P.380
http://www.ncbi.nlm.nih.gov/pmc/articles/PMC3583886/

HYDROFLUOCARBONS: HFC. Several organic compounds. Decreasingly used as refrigerants. P.5
https://www.britannica.com/science/hydrofluorocarbon

HYPERGLYCEMIA: Abnormally increased blood glucose levels. P.153, 158, 265
https://ccforum.biomedcentral.com/articles/10.1186/cc12514
http://joe.endocrinology-journals.org/content/204/1/1.full.pdf

HYPERPLASIA: Overgrowth of tissue. Increase in cellular reproduction rate. P.117, 137, 149
http://journals.lww.com/jaapa/Fulltext/2016/08000/

Benign_prostatic_hyperplasia__A_clinical_review.2.aspx
http://emedicine.medscape.com/article/269919-overview

HYPERTENSION: High blood pressure. Recently defined as 130 mm Hg systolic (pressure during heart muscle contraction), and 80 mm HG diastolic (pressure during relaxation). P.65, 73, 157, 282

http://jaha.ahajournals.org/content/4/12/e002315.full

http://www.jwatch.org/na43262/2017/03/02/pharmaco-logic-treatment-hypertension-older-adults?query=etoc_jwgenmed&jwd=000012066693&jspc=OBG

http://hyper.ahajournals.org/content/early/2017/11/10/HYP.0000000000000065

https://jamanetwork.com/journals/jama/fullarticle/2664350?utm_source=silverchair&utm_medium=email&utm_campaign=article_alert-jama&utm_content=olf&u

https://jamanetwork.com/journals/jama/fullarticle/2664350?&utm_source=191323&utm_medium=BulletinHealthCare&utm_term=120217&utm_content=Mornin

HYPOTENSION, ORTHOSTATIC: Low blood pressure on standing.
http://www.ncbi.nlm.nih.gov/pubmed/27225359?access_num=27225359&link_type=MED&dopt=Abstract

HYPOTHALAMUS: Part of the brain below the thalamus. Forms the major portion of the ventral region of the diencephalon. Forms part of the wall of the third

ventricle. P.186, 250, 284
http://press.endocrine.org/doi/abs/10.1210/jc.2015-2236

HYSTERECTOMY: Surgical removal of the uterus. P.148

HYSTEROSALPINGOGRAM: Injection of radiopaque dye into the uterus via the cervix to radiologically visualize the uterine cavity, the fallopian tubes, and their patency. P.245

HYSTEROSCOPY: A minimally invasive surgical technique in which a fiberoptic telescope (hysteroscope) is introduced through the cervical os into the uterine cavity. The endometrial lining of the uterus and the interior openings of the fallopian tubes can be seen. P.135, 146, 194, 245

ICSI: Intracytoplasmic sperm injection. P.29, 247, 248
http://americanpregnancy.org/infertility/intracytoplasmic-sperm-injection/

IMMUNE SYSTEM: The system that allows the body to ward off invasion by foreign substances, including infectious agents. Cells including T-lymphocytes that go to infected sites are elaborated in bone marrow and other areas. Antibodies (immunoglobulins) that target specific invaders (antigens) circulate in the bloodstream. Infected areas drain through lymphatic channels to the lymph nodes, where invading organisms are processed. P.45, 154, 249

http://emedicine.medscape.com/article
/1948753-overview

IMMUNOCYTE: Leukocyte that induces immune
response by antibody production in reaction to an
antigen. P.254
http://www.feinsteininstitute.org/programs-researchers
/immunology/immunocytes-cytokine-biology/

IMMUNOGLOBULIN: Ig. Proteins that function as antibodies and bind to antigens. P.297
http://www.ebioscience.com/knowledge-center/antigen
/immunoglobulin.htm

Frontiers | B Cell Intrinsic Mechanisms Constraining
IgE Memory | Immunology

IMMUNOSUPPRESSION: Suppression of the immune
response. P.45
http://emedicine.medscape.com/article/432316-overview

IMMUNOTHERAPY: Prevention or treatment of
disease with substances that stimulate the immune
response. Blocking the shut-off of the immune response.
Anticancer vaccines. P.116
https://www.mdanderson.org/treatment-options/immu-
notherapy.html
http://journal.frontiersin.org/article/10.3389/
fimmu.2016.00621/full?utm_source=newsletter&utm_
medium=email&utm_campaign=Immunology-w1-2017

http://journal.frontiersin.org/article/10.3389/
fimmu.2016.00621/full?utm_source=newsletter&utm_
medium=email&utm_campaign=Immunology-w1-2017
http://www.mdedge.com/jcso/article/135689/gastroen-
terology/meeting-potential-immunotherapy-new-targets-
provide-rational/pdf?channel=213
http://journal.frontiersin.org/article/10.3389/
fimmu.2017.00555/full?utm_source=F-AAE&utm_
medium=EMLF&utm_campaign=MRK_275249_35_
Immuno_20170518_arts_A
https://www.frontiersin.org/articles/10.3389/
fimmu.2018.00384/full?utm_source=F-AAE&utm_
medium=EMLF&utm_campaign=MRK_571163_35_

IMPLANTATION: The sperm fertilizes (fuses with) the egg (ovum) in the fallopian tube. The fertilized egg then migrates from the fallopian tube into the uterus at a specific time , when the endometrium is most receptive, and attaches to and burrows into the uterine lining.

IMPRINTING: (Genomic Imprinting) The process by which only the copy of a gene from one parent gets switched on in an offspring.
https://www.genome.gov/27532724/
https://ghr.nlm.nih.gov/primer/inheritance/
updimprinting

INDUCED PLURIPOTENT STEM CELLS: IPS. Cells from an adult human that have been reprogrammed into

an embryonic-like state.
http://stemcells.nih.gov/info/basics/pages/basics10.aspx
http://www.nature.com/news/japanese-man-is-first-
to-receive-reprogrammed-stem-cells-from-another-
person-1.21730?WT.ec_id=NEWS-20170330&spMailin-
gID=53740049&sp

INFARCT: Cutoff of blood supply causing tissue death,
resulting in a scarred area. P.9, 64, 65, 67, 83, 159, 196, 255
http://www.omicsonline.org/biomarkers-in-acute-myo-
cardial-infarction-2155-9880.1000222.pdf

INFECTION: Invasion of foreign organisms, such as bacteria or viruses, into the body. P. 4, 20, 24, 25, 36, 41, 42,
68, 236, 260, 261, 262, 264, 266, 267, 317, 356, 357, 385, 395
http://www.ph.ucla.edu/epi/faculty/detels/epi220/
detels_agents.pdf

INFLAMMATION: The body's response to infection or
injury, including redness, swelling, and heat. The specific
responses are geared to killing the infectious agent and
repairing the damaged tissue. P.154, 178, 249
http://journal.frontiersin.org/article/10.3389/
fimmu.2017.00017/full?utm_source=newsletter&utm_
medium=email&utm_campaign=Immunology-w4-2017

INFLUENZA: Contagious respiratory illness caused by
influenza virus. P.267
http://journals.lww.com/epidem/Abstract/2015/11000/

Review_Article___The_Fraction_of_Influenza_Virus.13.
aspx

http://www.cdc.gov/mmwr/volumes/65/rr/rr6505a1.htm

INFORMATION TECHNOLOGY: IT. Computerized
paperless data keeping, analysis, and transmission.
http://www.intel.com/content/www/us/en/healthcare-it
/collaborative-care.html?cid=sem43700013297809532&
intel_term=technology+for+healthcare&gclid=
Cj0KEQjw6am-BRCTk4WZhLfd4-oBEiQA3ydA3
IK6NZjCN51AIK72GMKucyGNX297Xgy6h66th96
XBwcaAhYO8P8HAQ&gclsrc=aw.ds

INHIBINS: Peptides made in granulosa cells of ovarian
follicles that inhibit secretion of follicle stimulating hormone (FSH). P.187, 192
http://www.medicinenet.com/script/main/art.asp?arti-
clekey=22571
http://press.endocrine.org/doi/abs/10.1210/
endo-124-1-552

INSOMNIA: Sleeplessness. P.218

INSULIN: Polypeptide hormone, produced by the beta
cells of the islets of Langerhans in the pancreas, that regulates blood glucose P.153
http://onlinelibrary.wiley.com/doi/10.1002/bip.20734/full

INSULIN RESISTANCE: Lowered level of response to insulin. P.289, 391
http://emedicine.medscape.com/article/122501-overview

INTERFERON: A protein that can inhibit virus replication. P.297, 391
https://www.drugs.com/drug-class/interferons.html
http://journal.frontiersin.org/article/10.3389/
fimmu.2017.00062/full?utm_source=newsletter&utm_
medium=email&utm_campaign=Immunology-w7-2017

INTERSTITIAL CYSTITIS: Painful Bladder Syndrome (BPS). P.236
http://emedicine.medscape.com/article
/2055505-overview

INTERSTITIAL SPACE: Small, narrow, fluid containing space between tissues
https://www.ncbi.nlm.nih.gov/pmc/articles/
PMC3139075/
https://www.thefreedictionary.com/interstitial+space

INTERSTITIUM: Fluid filled interstitial space draining to lymph nodes, supported by a network of collagen bundles. Visualized by laser endomicroscopy in relation to the extrahepatic bile duct, and other tissues that are subject to intermittent compression, including the submucosa of the gastrointestinal tract, and the urinary bladder.
https://www.nature.com/articles/s41598-018-23062-6

INTRAUTERINE ENVIRONMENT: The environment in which the growing fetus lives. P.240, 259

INTRAUTERINE GROWTH RETARDATION: IUGR. Fetal growth restriction. P.260
http://www.uptodate.com/contents/
fetal-growth-restriction-evaluation-and-management

ISCHEMIA: Inadequate blood supply to an organ, resulting in inadequate oxygenation. P.67

KAPOSI'S SARCOMA: Malignancy with cutaneous lesions caused by HHV8: human herpesvirus 8. Tends to occur in immunosuppressed individuals, notably those with AIDS (Autoimmune Deficiency Syndrome). P.263
http://emedicine.medscape.com/article/279734-overview

KERATOPLASTY: Conductive keratoplasty. CK. Eye surgery utilizing radio frequency energy to change the shape of the cornea. P. 387

KILLER CELL: Natural killer (**NK**) cells are derived from hematopoietic stem cells in bone marrow. They kill cancer cells by secreting **perforins** (cytolytic proteins) and **granzymes** (proteases : enzymes that catalyze degradation of protein)
https://www.ncbi.nlm.nih.gov/pmc/articles/
PMC4346487/
https://en.wikipedia.org/wiki/Granzyme
http://medical-dictionary.thefreedictionary.com/perforin

http://www.dictionary.com/browse/protease

http://journal.frontiersin.org/article/10.3389/
fimmu.2016.00492/full

http://journal.frontiersin.org/article/10.3389/
fimmu.2017.00293/full?utm_source=newsletter&utm_
medium=email&utm_campaign=Immunology-w12-2017

http://journal.frontiersin.org/article/10.3389/
fimmu.2017.00683/full?utm_source=F-AAE&utm_
medium=EMLF&utm_campaign=MRK_307979_35_
Immuno_20170622_arts_A

http://journal.frontiersin.org/article/10.3389/
fimmu.2017.00760/full?utm_source=F-AAE&utm_
medium=EMLF&utm_campaign=MRK_320984_35_
Immuno_20170706_arts_A

http://journal.frontiersin.org/article/10.3389/
fimmu.2017.00930/full?utm_source=F-AAE&utm_
medium=EMLF&utm_campaign=MRK_352999_35_
Immuno_20170808_arts_A

http://journal.frontiersin.org/article/10.3389/
fimmu.2017.00774/full?utm_source=F-AAE&utm_
medium=EMLF&utm_campaign=MRK_333189_35_
Immuno_20170720_arts_A

http://journal.frontiersin.org/article/10.3389/
fimmu.2017.01061/full?utm_source=F-AAE&utm_
medium=EMLF&utm_campaign=MRK_398354_35_
Immuno_20170921_arts_A

KINASE: Enzyme important in the carbohydrate metabolism and energy output of cells. Protein-Tyrosine Kinases (PTK's) regulate signaling in the cell. If PTK signaling is disrupted, malignant transformation of the cell can result. P.66
http://www.ncbi.nlm.nih.gov/pubmed/10966463
http://www.sciencedirect.com/science/article/pii/S1043661813001771

LABOR: Period from the onset of regular uterine contractions with dilatation and effacement of the cervix and descent of the fetus through the birth canal culminating in delivery of the baby. P.232, 260

LACTIC ACIDOSIS: Increased plasma lactate. P.159. See: The Care of the Older Person: How To Diagnose And Treat Delirium : Haiban Yin.
http://emedicine.medscape.com/article/167027-overview

LACTOSE INTOLERANCE: Inability to digest lactose, a disaccharide in milk made up of glucose and galactose. P.281
http://emedicine.medscape.com/article/187249-overview

LAPAROSCOPY: a minimally invasive surgical technique in which a fiberoptic telescope (laparoscope) is introduced into the abdominal cavity through a small incision near the lower margin of the umbilicus. P. XIII, 120, 143, 245, 246, 250, 269

LASER: Light Amplification by Stimulated Emission of Radiation. A narrow, often powerful, beam of light which does not spread and is monochromatic. This is a directed light beam, not nuclear radiation. P.3, 250, 381, 393
http://www.azooptics.com/Article.aspx?ArticleID=44
http://www.nature.com/articles/s41551-016-0008?
WT.mc_id=EMI_NBME_1701_LAUNCHISSUE_
PORTFOLIO&spMailingID=53217285&spUserID=MTc3
MDI4ODk5NQS2&spJobID=1083253126&spReportId=
MTA4MzI1MzEyNgS2

LEPTIN: Hormone produced by adipocytes involved in fat storage regulation. Acts on hypothalamus to suppress appetite. P.284
http://www.sciencedirect.com/science/article/pii/
S0083672905710128

LEUKEMIA: Malignant form of white blood cells in the blood stream, commonly arising from the bone marrow.
http://www.ncbi.nlm.nih.gov/pmc/articles/PMC3396664/

LIBIDO: Sexual drive. P.204, 221, 222
https://en.wikipedia.org/wiki/Flibanserin
http://www.medscape.com/viewarticle/871481?
nlid=110609_2581&src=WNL_mdplsnews_161111_msc-
pedit_obgy&uac=66536PR&spon=16&impID=1232827&
faf=1

LIFE EXPECTANCY: The age to which an individual or a selected population group might live. See: The Care of The Older Person : Introduction: Jose Morais. P. 257-274, ix-xvii, 1-49.

https://www.zionmarketresearch.com/report/home-healthcare-markethttp://science.sciencemag.org/content/360/6396/1459

http://onlinelibrary.wiley.com/doi/10.1002/sres.2420/full
http://www.cdc.gov/nchs/data/hus/2011/022.pdf
http://www.statcan.gc.ca/tables-tableaux/sum-som/l01/cst01/health26-eng.htm
http://www.cdc.gov/nchs/data/databriefs/db267.pdf
http://mdlinx.pdr.net/internal-medicine/news-article.cfm/6986115/?utm_source=in-house&utm_medium=message&utm_campaign=mh-im-dec16
http://journals.plos.org/plosbiology/article?id=10.1371/journal.pbio.2002458#pbio.2002458.ref039

LIPOSUCTION: Surgical removal of fat by suction. P.378, 382, 383

LIQUID BIOPSY: Blood testing for circulating tumor DNA (ctDNA). Identifies cancer mutations useful as biomarkers, many associated with targeted drug.
http://www.ncbi.nlm.nih.gov/pmc/articles/PMC4356857/
http://www.nature.com/nrclinonc/posters/liquidbiopsies/nrclinonc_liquidbiopsies_poster_web.pdf
http://www.nature.com/news/

liquid-biopsies-success-highlights-power-of-combin-
ing-basic-and-clinical-research-1.21883?WT.ec_id=
NATURE-20170427&spMailingID=53937339&
https://www.nature.com/articles/s41551-017-0065?WT.
mc_id=EMI_NBME_1704_APRILISSUE_PORTFOLIO&
spMailingID=53957850&spUserID=MTc3MDI4ODk5NQS

LOW DENSITY LIPOPROTEIN: LDL. Complex of lipids and proteins that transports cholesterol in the blood.
Significant factor in the formation of arteriosclerotic
plaques. P.77 154, 201, 298
http://www.ncbi.nlm.nih.gov/pubmed/10073963

LUNG CANCER: Malignant tumor in the lung. Major
cause of cancer deaths. Predominant type is Non- Small
Cell Lung Cancer (**NSCLC**), strongly linked to tobacco
smoking.
https://cancerstaging.org/references-tools/quickrefer-
ences/Documents/LungMedium.pdf
https://www.ncbi.nlm.nih.gov/pmc/articles/
PMC3864624/
https://www.ncbi.nlm.nih.gov/pmc/articles/
PMC4367711/
https://www.ncbi.nlm.nih.gov/pmc/articles/
PMC5107578/
http://www.jtcvsonline.org/article/S0022-5223(17)31171-6
/fulltext#sec1.6

LUTEINIZING HORMONE: LH. Secreted by the anterior pituitary, surges prior to ovulation. Acts on the ovary P.186, 188, 192, 244, 245, 250
http://emedicine.medscape.com/article
/2089268-overview

LYME DISEASE: Tick-borne illness caused by Borrelia burgdorferi. Other tick-borne illnesses include babesiosis, anaplasmosis, ehrlichosis, and Rocky Mountain Spotted Fever. P. 319
http://www.ncbi.nlm.nih.gov/pmc/articles/PMC3542482/

LYMPH NODE: Small and bean shaped, lymph nodes are present throughout the body. They are composed of lymphoid tissue, and are connected by lymph channels. The lymphatic system is important in the immune response, in fighting infection. Cancerous cells can enter the lymphatic system and drain to lymph nodes, enlarging them. Cancer surgery often involves the removal of affected lymph nodes, or lymph nodes that are likely to be affected by a cancer. P.253
https://www.boundless.com/physiology/textbooks/
boundless-anatomy-and-physiology-textbook/lymphatic-
system-20/lymph-cells-and-tissues-193/lymph-nodes-
963-3100/

LYMPHOCYTE: A form of white blood cell. B cells and T cells are two main types. P.253, 269

http://www.ncbi.nlm.nih.gov/pubmedhealth/
PMHT0022042/

LYMPHOMA: A solid malignant tumor often composed
of cells that resemble lymphocytes. Can arise at various
sites within the body and invade the bloodstream.
http://www.bloodjournal.org/content/125/1/22

LYNCH SYNDROME: Autosomal dominant inherited
predisposition for colon and endometrial cancers
https://www.ncbi.nlm.nih.gov/pmc/articles/
PMC2933058/
https://www.sgo.org/wp-content/uploads/2016/10/2016-
SGO-Genetics-Toolkit3.pdf

LYSOSOMES: Organelles in the cell containing enzymes
that degrade biologic polymers including proteins, car-
bohydrates and lipids.
https://www.ncbi.nlm.nih.gov/books/NBK9953/

MACROPHAGE: A large phagocytic white blood cell.
P.253
http://www.cell.com/immunity/fulltext/
S1074-7613(14)00235-0

MACULAR DEGENERATION: Deterioration of the
macula, the area surrounding the fovea near the center
of the retina in the eye. P.389
https://www.ncbi.nlm.nih.gov/pmc/articles/
PMC3732788/

https://www.nature.com/articles/nbt.4114.epdf?referrer_
access_token=8BtrAvy5kx0RIQxVHmwBfNRgN0jAjWeI-
9jnR3ZoTv0PJSqIFs8CVMGLKXeHOLTvVGIDHNZm

MALNUTRITION: Improper intake and processing
of foodstuffs. P.4, 54 See: The Care of the Older Person:
Could My Patient Be Malnourished? Jose A. Morais
https://www.ncbi.nlm.nih.gov/pubmed/16782522

MAMMOGRAPHY: Xray breast imaging. P.111, 330
http://emedicine.medscape.com/article/346529-overview
http://www.jwatch.org/na42993/2016/12/13/when-stop-
surveillance-mammography-older-breast-cancer?query=
etoc_jwwomen&jwd=000012066693&jspc=OBG

MAO INHIBITORS: Monoamine oxidase inhibitors,
sometimes still used in the treatment of depression.
Monoamine oxidase enzymes catalase oxidation and
inactivation of monoamine neurotransmitters , including
dopamine, noradrenaline, adrenaline and serotonin. P.216
http://www.webmd.com/depression/symptoms-
depressed-anxiety-12/antidepressants

MEDIASTINUM: Space in the thorax between the pleural sacs, notably containing the heart and its great vessels.
P.264
https://www.youtube.com/watch?v=2POIlBe2xR4

MEIOSIS: Cell division resulting in cells (gam-
etes) with a single set of chromosomes, half the

number of chromosomes present in the parent cell.
https://www.khanacademy.org/science/biology/
cellular-molecular-biology/meiosis/a/phases-of-meiosis

MELANOMA: Tumor of melanin-forming cells. P.390
http://www.medicaljournals.se/acta/content/?
doi=10.2340/00015555-2035&html=1
https://www.cell.com/cell/fulltext/S0092-8674(17)30952-2

MENOPAUSE: Cessation of menses. P.134, 145, 148, 185, 187, 226, 327
https://www.ncbi.nlm.nih.gov/pmc/articles/
PMC3285482/

MENSTRUATION: Blood and shedding endometrium from the uterus beginning approximately fourteen days after ovulation in a non-pregnant cycle. P.248, 249, 250
https://www.ncbi.nlm.nih.gov/pubmed/16160098

METABOLIC ACIDOSIS: Increase in plasma acidity. Excess production of acid with inadequate buffer, bicarbonate, to neutralize it. Insufficient renal excretion of acid. P.197
http://www.nature.com/nrneph/journal/v6/n5/abs/
nrneph.2010.33.html

METABOLIC SYNDROME: Central (abdominal)obesity, hypertension, and insulin resistance. High levels of triglycerides, low levels of HDL. P.156, 178
http://www.ncbi.nlm.nih.gov/pmc/articles/PMC3966331/

METABOLISM: Molecular chemical reactions within living tissue. P.35, 291
http://www.biology-pages.info/C/CellularRespiration.html

METAPLASIA: A benign cell change. In a common type, glandular epithelium is transformed into squamous epithelium. P.132, 133
https://en.wikipedia.org/wiki/Squamous_metaplasia

METFORMIN: Oral anti-hyperglycemic agent used
https://www.ncbi.nlm.nih.gov/pubmed/29800211in
Type 2 Diabetes. Decreases hepatic glucose production. Implications in other disease states, weight loss, and possibly lifespan.
https://www.ncbi.nlm.nih.gov/pmc/articles/
PMC3398862/

MICROBIOME: Bacteria that inhabit the gut.
http://jamanetwork.com/journals/jama/fullarticle
/2594788

MICROGLIA: Immune, phagocytic, central nervous system (brain and spinal cord) cells implicated in Alzheimer's Disease
https://www.sciencedirect.com/science/article/pii/
S0896627300801877#!
https://www.ncbi.nlm.nih.gov/pubmed/17504139

https://www.nature.com/articles/d41586-018-04930-
7?utm_source=briefing-dy&utm_medium=email&utm_
campaign=briefing&utm_content=20180425

MICROSURGERY: Surgery performed with visualization through a microscope, often involving anastomoses
of small blood vessels. P.166

MIGRAINE: Vascular headaches involving the blood vessels of the brain. P.195
http://www.ncbi.nlm.nih.gov/pmc/articles/PMC3663475/
https://www.jwatch.org/fw113584/2017/11/30/migraine-
prevention-two-calcitonin-gene-related-peptide?query=
pfwTOC&jwd=000012066693&jspc=OBG
http://www.pdr.net/drug-summary/
Imitrex-Tablets-sumatriptan-succinate-201
https://www.ncbi.nlm.nih.gov/pubmed/29800211

MITOCHONDRIA: Intracellular organelle in which respiration and energy production occur. P.157
http://citeseerx.ist.psu.edu/viewdoc/download?
doi=10.1.1.572.8830&rep=rep1&type=pdf
http://www.cell.com/cell-metabolism/fulltext/S1550-
4131(16)30502-2
http://mdlinx.pdr.net/neurology/news-article.cfm
/6907659?utm_source=in-house&utm_medium=mes-
sage&utm_campaign=medhead
https://link.springer.com/article/10.1007/

s10815-017-1006-3/fulltext.html?wt_mc=alerts.
TOCjournals
https://www.deepdyve.com/lp/springer-journal/quan-
titative-and-qualitative-changes-of-mitochondria-in-
human-Gh20vR9aBa?key=bioportfolio

MITOSIS: Cell division resulting in daughter cells identical to the parent cell. https://www.khanacademy.org/
science/biology/cellular-molecular-biology/meiosis/a/
phases-of-meiosis

MOBILITY: Ability to move freely and easily. See The
Care of the Older Person: Why Does My Patient Have
Gait and Balance Disorders? : Olivier Beauchet
https://www.mayoclinic.org/diseases-conditions/move-
ment-disorders/symptoms-causes/syc-20363893
https://en.oxforddictionaries.com/definition/mobility

MOHS SURGERY: Surgery in which thin layers of cancer containing skin are stepwise removed and examined
microscopically, until only cancer free tissue remains.
P.390
http://emedicine.medscape.com/article/2212475-overview

MONOCLONAL ANTIBODY: An antibody that will go
to a specific receptor site. "Monoclonal" refers to the fact
that the antibody protein is derived from one clone of

cells, all of which are identical. P.95, 101, 167
http://www.ncbi.nlm.nih.gov/pmc/articles/PMC4491443/

MONTREAL COGNITIVE ASSESSMENT: MoCA: Test
to detect mild cognitive impairment and Alzheimer's
disease. The Care of the Older Person: Chapt: "Doctor,
my wife is getting forgetful": Serge Gauthier
**http://dementia.ie/images/uploads/site-images/MoCA-
Test-English_7_1.pdf**
http://www.mocatest.org/

**https://www.sciencedirect.com/topics/neuroscience/
montreal-cognitive-assessment**

MRI: Magnetic Resonance Imaging. An advanced
imaging technique that uses a powerful magnet to
alter polarity. P.35, 98, 112, 137, 142, 147, 175, 244 https://
onlinelibrary.wiley.com/doi/full/10.1002/jmri.23642

MSG: Monosodium glutamate. P.196
http://www.mayoclinic.org/healthy-lifestyle/nutrition-
and-healthy-eating/expert-answers/monosodium-gluta-
mate/faq-20058196

MOTORIC COGNITIVE RISK SYNDROME (MCR):
Predementia syndrome combining cognitive complaint
and slow gait.

http://biomedgerontology.oxfordjournals.org/content
/71/8/1081

MULTIPLE MYELOMA: Plasma cell (a type of white
blood cell derived from B cell) malignancy. Anemia
and osteolytic (bone reabsorbing) skeletal lesions usually present. A monoclonal (M) protein can usually be
detected in the blood serum and urine.
https://www.mdedge.com/oncologypractice/article
/154492/multiple-myeloma/crb-410-update-multiple-
myeloma-response-rates?oc_slh=1de3dcf7eb6395af6
b796baf8538c
https://www.ncbi.nlm.nih.gov/pmc/articles/
PMC5223450/
https://www.cancer.gov/publications/dictionaries/can-
cer-terms?cdrid=46230
https://www.cancer.gov/publications/dictionaries/can-
cer-terms?cdrid=45810

MUTATION: Abnormal recombinations of the chromosomes. Alteration in a genome, that may or may not be
harmful to the individual. P, VIII, 18, 173
http://www.nature.com/scitable/definition/recombina-
tion-226
http://www.ncbi.nlm.nih.gov/pubmed/23266571

MYELIN: Insulating sheath around nerve fibers. P.169
http://www.news-medical.net/health/Myelin-Function.
aspx

MYELODYSPLASIA (MDS): Syndromes of bone marrow failure
http://www.mdedge.com/jcso/article/118728/leukemia-myelodysplasia-transplantation/myelodysplastic-syndromes-etiologies?channel=238&utm_source=News_OP-JCSO_enl_121716&utm_medium=email&utm_content=Myelodysplastic%20syndromes:%20etiologies,%20evaluation,%20and%20therapy

MYELOPEROXIDASE: MPO. Enzyme in neutrophils linked to cardiovascular disease. P.63, 64
http://www.ncbi.nlm.nih.gov/gene/4353
http://www.ncbi.nlm.nih.gov/pubmed/26567811/

MYOCARDIAL INFARCTION: Irreversible injury to heart muscle. P.9, 64, 65, 67, 83, 159, 178, 212
http://www.clevelandclinicmeded.com/medicalpubs/diseasemanagement/cardiology/acute-myocardial-infarction/
https://arxiv.org/abs/1708.09843

MYOCARDIUM: Heart muscle.
https://www.boundless.com/physiology/textbooks/boundless-anatomy-and-physiology-textbook/

cardiovascular-system-the-heart-18/the-heart-172/myo-cardial-thickness-and-function-867-10251/

MYOCYTE: Heart muscle cell. P.46, 64, 71
https://www.sciencedaily.com/releases/2016/04
/160421145756.htm

MYOMECTOMY: Surgical removal of fibroids from the uterus. P.146, 147

NANOTECHNOLOGY: Engineering of tiny machines, often for the monitoring, prevention, and treatment of disease. P.36, 39
http://tedx.tumblr.com/post/35204848311/fight-cancer-with-nanotechnology-sylvain-martel
http://iopscience.iop.org/journal/0957-4484;jses-sionid=3420F74BB331365A7161E71B24C8121C.c4.iop-science.cld.iop.org
http://journal.frontiersin.org/article/10.3389/
fimmu.2017.00069/full?utm_source=newsletter&utm_medium=email&utm_campaign=Immunology-w6-2017
https://www.nature.com/articles/s41551-017-0029?
WT.mc_id=LDN_NBME_1801_FIRSTANNIVERSARY_
PORTFOLIO

NARRATIVE MEDICINE: Narrative competence: Listening to and understanding related stories , and appropriately responding.
http://www.ncbi.nlm.nih.gov/pmc/articles/PMC3034473/

NEPHROPATHY: Kidney disease or damage. P.265
http://www.ncbi.nlm.nih.gov/pmc/articles/PMC3084647/
https://en.wikipedia.org/wiki/Kidney_disease

NEPHROSIS: Generally refers to degenerative disease of the renal (kidney) tubules
http://medical-dictionary.thefreedictionary.com/nephrosis

NEPHROTIC SYNDROME: Excretion of significant amounts of protein in the urine, along with decreased serum albumin (a protein), and edema (swelling due to fluid accumulation)
http://emedicine.medscape.com/article/244631-overview

NEURAL TUBE DEFECT: Birth defect of brain, spine, or spinal cord. P.298
http://www.ncbi.nlm.nih.gov/pmc/articles/PMC4023229/

NEUROGENESIS: Formation of neurons
https://www.nature.com/articles/nature25975

NEUROIMMUNE COMMUNICATION: Interaction between the nervous and immune systems, influencing each other.
http://www.nature.com/ni/journal/v18/n2/full/ni.3676.html
http://www.nature.com/neuro/journal/v20/n2/full/nn.4496.html

NEUROMORPHIC ENGINEERING: Designing hardware and physical models of neural and sensory systems. https://www.frontiersin.org/journals/neuroscience/sections/neuromorphic-engineering http://compneuro.uwaterloo.ca/research/nef/overview-of-the-nef.html

NEURON: Specialized nervous system cell that can be stimulated and conducts impulses. P.41, 46, 85 http://www.ncbi.nlm.nih.gov/books/NBK21535/

NEUTROPHIL: A white blood cell containing granules that are enzyme containing sacs. P.267 http://jem.rupress.org/content/210/7/1283.full

NICOTINAMIDE RIBOSIDE: NR: A form of Vitamin B3 (nicotinic acid, Niacin). Converts to **NAD,** Nicotinamide Adenine Dinucleotide, a coenzyme in cells that is involved in energy metabolism

http://www.ctl.cornell.edu/events/ctvf12/Sauve.pdf http://jpet.aspetjournals.org/content/324/3/883.full

NITRITES: Ester or salt of nitrous acid. Vasodilator. P.196 http://circ.ahajournals.org/content/117/16/2151

NUCLEAR POWER: Energy produced by atomic reaction. P.5 http://www.nei.org/Knowledge-Center/How-Nuclear-Reactors-Work

NUCLEAR WASTE: Radioactive byproducts usually from operation of a nuclear reactor.
http://www.nrc.gov/reading-rm/doc-collections/fact-sheets/radwaste.html
http://www.nrc.gov/reading-rm/doc-collections/fact-sheets/radwaste.html

NUCLEASE: Enzyme that catalyzes the cleavage of phosphodiester bonds between nucleotides.
http://www.nature.com/onc/journal/v21/n58/full/1206135a.html?foxtrotcallback=true
https://www.ncbi.nlm.nih.gov/pubmed/24690881
https://www.ncbi.nlm.nih.gov/pubmed/24690881

NUCLEIC ACID: Substance found in the cytoplasm of cells, as well as in chromosomes, and in viruses. Four specific nucleic acids: adenine (A), cytosine (C), guanine (G), and thymine (T) are arranged in pairs on each rung of the ladder of DNA. They code the sequences of amino acids that make up proteins. P.34
http://www.rsc.org/Education/Teachers/Resources/cfb/nucleicacids.htm

NUCLEOSOME: The basic structural unit of chromatin.
https://en.wikipedia.org/wiki/Chromatin
https://www.nature.com/scitable/topicpage/dna-packaging-nucleosomes-and-chromatin-310

NUCLEOTIDE: Building block (subunit) of nucleic acid. Nitrogenous base plus ribose or deoxyribose plus one or more phosphate groups.

https://en.wikipedia.org/wiki/Nucleotide

NUCLEUS: A central structure, surrounded by its own membrane, in the cell. The nucleus contains the chromosomes. P.32, 41

https://micro.magnet.fsu.edu/cells/nucleus/nucleus.html
https://micro.magnet.fsu.edu/cells/nucleus/nucleus.html

NURSING: Breastfeeding. P.356

OBESITY: More than 20% above expected body weight, Body Mass Index (BMI) of 30 or more. P.4, 9, 11, 65, 74, 78, 107, 153, 154, 157, 282, 290, 327

http://www.ncbi.nlm.nih.gov/pubmed/22171945
https://www.ncbi.nlm.nih.gov/pubmed/27386756
http://www.cell.com/cell/fulltext/S0092-8674(16)30213-6
https://www.frontiersin.org/articles/10.3389/
fimmu.2017.01745/full?utm_source=F-AAE&utm_
medium=EMLF&utm_campaign=MRK_491010_35_I

ONCOLOGIST: Physician who specializes in the treatment of cancer.

http://www.oncologypractice.com/jcso/specialty-focus
/lung/single-article-page/genomic-oncology-moving-
beyond-the-tip-of-the-iceberg/0a952f61278bdd07e9d7db4
e7c6d1fcb.html

OPHTHALMIC NERVE: Branch of the trigeminal nerve that gives sensory fibers to the ciliary muscle of the eye, lacrimal gland, eyelids, forehead, and mucous membrane of the nose. P.195

http://www.ncbi.nlm.nih.gov/pubmed/11842844

OPIOID: Naturally occurring and synthetic potentially addictive substances that act on specific (opioid) receptors to produce effects including pain relief. Major cause of drug abuse, addiction, and death.

https://www.drugabuse.gov/drugs-abuse/opioids
https://www.drugabuse.gov/drugs-abuse/opioids/opioid-crisis
https://www.fda.gov/Drugs/DrugSafety/InformationbyDrugClass/ucm337066.htm

OSTEOBLAST: Cell that synthesizes bone. P.207
www.nature.com/articles/boneres20169

OSTEOCLAST: Cell that reabsorbs bone. P.207, 210
http://www.ncbi.nlm.nih.gov/pubmed/1873485

OSTEOPENIA: Reduced bone mass. Less severe than osteoporosis. P.327
medicine.medscape.com/article/330598-overview

OSTEOPOROSIS: Reduced bone mass due to depletion of calcium and bone protein. P.206, 278
https://www.karger.com/Article/FullText/431091
http://www.thelancet.com/journals/lancet/article/

PIIS0140-6736(17)31613-6/fulltext
https://mydigimag.rrd.com/publication/?i=470718&ver=
html5&p=30&utm_source=PT+eTOC+2018-02+prospect+
no+spons&utm_campaign=PT1802_Digital_Edition_
Alert&utm_medium=email#{"page":"30"

OVARIAN CANCER: Cancer of the ovary.
https://www.ncbi.nlm.nih.gov/pmc/articles/PMC5365187/
https://www.uptodate.com/contents/
screening-for-ovarian-cancer

OVARY: The primary female sex organ. Almond shaped,
3 centimeters long. Two ovaries, one on either side of the
uterus in the pelvis. P.247, 248
http://emedicine.medscape.com/article/1949171-overview
http://www.fertstert.org/article/S0015-0282(17)31879-4
/fulltext?elsca1=etoc&elsca2=email&
elsca3=0015-0282_201710_108_4_&elsca4=
Obstetrics%20and%20Gyn

OVULATION: During the menstrual cycle, several fluid
filled follicles, each containing an ovum, develop. One
becomes the dominant follicle. The other follicles regress.
At midcycle, the dominant follicle ruptures, releasing the
egg, which is then picked up by the fimbria of the fallopian tube. P. 245, 247
https://www.ncbi.nlm.nih.gov/books/NBK279054/

OVUM: Pleural: ova. The oocyte. The egg. A single cell present in the female ovary that eventually can be fertilized by a single sperm cell from the male. The ovum before fertilization has only twenty three chromosomes. These pair with the twenty three chromosomes from the spermatozoon to create a genetically new individual with forty six chromosomes. P.44, 247, 248, 253

http://www.theodora.com/anatomy/the_ovum.html

PALLIATIVE CARE: Team support system of enhanced physical, psychosocial , and spiritual quality of life in the face of life-threatening illness. Prevention and relief of suffering and pain. Affirmation of life, and regarding dying as a normal process.

http://www.who.int/cancer/palliative/definition/en/

PAPANICOLAOU SMEAR: Cells in cervical mucus examined microscopically . P.XII, 121, 127, 135, 328, 331

https://www.google.com/search?q=photographs+
of+normal+and+ascus+cells&rlz=1C1CHBF_enUS694
US694&espv=2&biw=1745&bih=883&tbm=isch&tbo=
u&source=univ&sa=X&ved=0ahUKEwittZaMp57
PAhUELyYKHeGjBJcQsAQIGw

PARATHYROID HORMONE: PTH. Secreted by parathyroid glands. Regulates blood levels of calcium and phosphorus. P.210

http://www.ncbi.nlm.nih.gov/pubmed/19395963

PARKINSONISM: Parkinson disease. Chronic progressive debilitating neurologic condition arising in the basal ganglia of the brain. Loss of dopaminergic cells. Decreased dopamine production in substantia nigra. The Care of the Older Person: Why Does My Patient Have Gait & Balance Disorders? : Olivier Beauchet. P.179, 266
http://www.neurobiologyofaging.org/article/S0197-4580(16)30060-4/abstract
https://www.nature.com/articles/s41531-017-0015-3?WT.mc_id_EMI_PARKD_1708_PMC&WT.ec_id=INTERNAL&spMailingID=54985332&spUserID=MTc3MDI4ODk

PATHOLOGIST: Physician specializing in the diagnosis of disease by inspecting organs and tumors, both by direct vision and microscopically.

PCI: Percutaneous coronary intervention. Coronary angioplasty. Stent introduced by catheter and placed in coronary artery. P.81
http://emedicine.medscape.com/article/161446-overview
http://emedicine.medscape.com/article/161446-technique

PEPTIDE: Two or more amino acids linked together.
https://www2.chemistry.msu.edu/faculty/reusch/virttx-tjml/protein2.htm

PERIMENOPAUSE: The time shortly before menopause. P.191

PERIPHERAL ARTERY OCCLUSIVE DISEASE:
Narrowing and blockage of smaller arteries. P.88
http://emedicine.medscape.com/article/460178-overview

PERSONALITY TYPE: Psychologic classification of individuals. P.358
http://mbtitoday.org/carl-jung-psychological-type/

PESSARY: Device placed in the vagina for support. P.239

PET SCAN: Positron Emission Tomography. The person being imaged is given sugar, which is tagged by radioactive isotope. Malignant cells tend to metabolize sugar at a higher rate, because they are actively growing and dividing. The increased radioactive uptake measured at a given site in the body infers that there may be a malignant tumor at that site. P.35, 98, 144, 174
http://journals.lww.com/thoracicimaging/Fulltext/2013/01000/Overview_of_Positron_Emission_Tomography,_Hybrid.4.aspx

PHAGOCYTOSIS: The engulfing of a cell fragment or foreign body by a cell.

http://www.dictionary.com/browse/phagocytosis

PHEROMONE: Chemical substance released by an individual that stimulates the behavior of other individuals. P.222

http://www.scientificamerican.com/article/are-human-pheromones-real/

PHLEBITIS: Inflammation of the walls of a vein. P.203
http://emedicine.medscape.com/article/463256-overview

PHYTOESTROGENS: Naturally occuring estrogen like compounds in plants. P.212
http://www.ncbi.nlm.nih.gov/pmc/articles/PMC3074428/

PITUITARY GLAND: Endocrine gland attached to the base of the brain that secretes hormones that act on other endocrine glands. P.192, 244, 250
http://teachmeanatomy.info/neuro/structures/pituitary-gland/

PLACENTA: Disc-shaped organ that forms in pregnancy, nourishes and supports the developing fetus, and secretes hormones. The surface that is in contact with the mother's uterine wall is composed of many tiny villi. The fetal blood circulates within these villi, which are bathed on their outside by maternal blood from arteries in the uterine wall. Exchange between mother and fetus of nutrients, waste products of metabolism, oxygen and carbon dioxide continuously occurs through the external lining of each villus. After the baby is delivered, the placenta detaches from the wall of the uterus, and is itself delivered. P.251, 260

https://www.nichd.nih.gov/about/meetings/2014/
Documents/BurtonWashington2014.pdf

PLASMA (BLOOD): Fluid part of the blood that carries
the blood cells
https://www.ncbi.nlm.nih.gov/pubmedhealth/
PMHT0022021/

PLASMID: Circular molecule of DNA found in bacteria.
https://www.nature.com/scitable/definition/
plasmid-plasmids-28

PLATELET: Cell fragment in blood involved in blood
clotting. P.67, 212
https://www.ouhsc.edu/platelets/platelets/platelets%20
intro.html

PMDD: Premenstrual dysphoric disorder. Premenstrual
mood and behavioral changes. P.193

PMS: Premenstrual syndrome. Various symptoms just
prior to, or with the onset of, a period. May include
depression, anxiety, bloating, constipation, diarrhea,
breast tenderness, weight gain, and headache. P.193

PNEUMONIA: Lung inflammation with congestion. P.262,
267, 268
https://www.ncbi.nlm.nih.gov/pmc/articles/PMC4072047/
https://www.ncbi.nlm.nih.gov/pmc/articles/PMC4072047/
https://www.ncbi.nlm.nih.gov/pmc/articles/PMC4072047/

POLAR BODY: Small cells resulting from two meiotic divisions of the oocyte. Contain the same DNA as the oocyte. P.29
http://www.ncbi.nlm.nih.gov/pmc/articles/PMC3164815/

POLLUTION: Presence in, or introduction into, the environment of harmful substances. P.4, 5

POLYP: Benign growth arising from a stalk. Polyps occur in the interior of the uterus , and may protrude out the cervical os. Polyps in the large intestine may be malignant. Polyps can grow on the vocal cords, and other areas.

POLYPHARMACY: Simultaneous use of multiple drugs, more than are medically necessary. See: The Care of the Older Person: Polypharmacy and Deprescribing in the Elderly: Louise Mallet
https://www.ncbi.nlm.nih.gov/pmc/articles/PMC3864987/

POSTMENOPAUSAL BLEEDING: Vaginal bleeding occurring after the menopause. P.194
https://www.ncbi.nlm.nih.gov/pmc/articles/PMC3951032/

PRECISION MEDICINE: Identification of the specific mutations in a tumor, so that targeted therapy can be brought to bear.
http://stm.sciencemag.org/content/7/300/300ps17.full

PREIMPLANTATION GENETIC DIAGNOSIS: PGD. Chromosomal analysis of the polar body (See: Polar body), or of a single embryonic cell.   P.27, 48, 174
http://emedicine.medscape.com/article/273415-overview

PRETERM INFANT: Formerly called prematurity. A baby born before thirty eight weeks of intrauterine life.
http://www.adelaide.edu.au/news/news88982.html

PROBIOTICS: Microorganisms, usually bacteria, with health benefits.   P.296
http://www.medicinenet.com/script/main/art.asp?articlekey=11901

PROGENITOR CELL: Activated in tissue repair; differentiate to replace damaged tissue. If signal to differentiate not processed, progenitor cells can keep on reproducing, leading to mutations
http://stemcell.childrenshospital.org/about-stem-cells/adult-somatic-stem-cells-101/what-are-progenitor-cells/

PROGESTERONE: A female sex hormone, made in the ovary, prominent in the second half of the menstrual cycle.   P.188, 201, 244, 250 253, 394
https://en.wikipedia.org/wiki/Progesterone

PROGESTIN: A progesterone-like substance.

PROGRAMMED CELL DEATH: See Apoptosis for references

PROKARYOTE: Single celled organism without a distinct nucleus , and no specialized organelles (except ribosomes). Includes Bacteria.
http://www.dictionary.com/browse/prokaryote

PROLACTIN: Hormone secreted by the anterior pituitary that stimulates lactation, P.244
http://www.ncbi.nlm.nih.gov/pubmed/11015620

PROLAPSE: Downward displacement of an organ. P.234, 238, 239
http://emedicine.medscape.com/article/276259-overview

PROSTAGLANDINS: Group of fatty acids that stimulate contractility of uterine and other smooth muscle. P.190
http://www.ncbi.nlm.nih.gov/pmc/articles/PMC3081099/

PROSTATE: Gland located below the bladder and surrounding the urethra in males. Prostatic fluid is secreted via ducts that open into the urethra.
http://www.ncbi.nlm.nih.gov/pubmedhealth/
PMH0072475/
http://www.ncbi.nlm.nih.gov/pmc/articles/PMC4633657/
http://jamanetwork.com/journals/jama/fullarticle/2618352?utm_medium=alert&utm_source=
JAMAPublishAheadofPrint&utm_campaign=11-04-2017

PROSTATE CANCER: Cancer of the prostate gland.
https://www.ncbi.nlm.nih.gov/pubmed/28655021

http://www.nejm.org/doi/full/10.1056/NEJMoa1715546?
query=main_nav_lg

PROTEIN: A specific sequence of amino acids. Specific
proteins are elaborated by specific genes. Proteins have
vital functions within the body. They make up the
structure of various organs, and are involved in their
function. They make up the hormones, and the enzymes
which facilitate chemical reactions in the body. They are
involved in immune response. P.34
https://en.wikipedia.org/wiki/Proteome

PROTEOMICS: The study of all the proteins in the body,
how they function and interact.. P. 38, 140.
http://proteomics.cancer.gov/whatisproteomics

PROTON PUMP INHIBITORS: Drugs that inhibit acid
secretion by gastric parietal cells. Used in gastroesophageal reflux disease (**GERD**).
https://www.ncbi.nlm.nih.gov/pmc/articles/PMC5221858/

PTK: Protein-tyrosine kinase. Regulates signaling in the
cell. P.105
http://www.ncbi.nlm.nih.gov/pubmed/9393984

PULMONARY EMBOLUS: PE. Blood clot in the lung. P.89
http://emedicine.medscape.com/article/300901-overview

RADIATION: Emission of energy as electromagnetic
waves or as moving subatomic particles, especially high

energy particles that cause ionization. Ionizing radiation has enough energy to remove electrons from the orbit of an atom, causing the atom to be charged (ionized). P.357, 396 http://www.who.int/ionizing_radiation/about/what_is_ir /en/

RECEPTOR SITE: Distinctively shaped area on a cell surface, designed to receive a specific substance. P.39, 66, 247, 250 http://www.merckmanuals.com/professional/clinical-pharmacology/pharmacodynamics/drug%E2%80%93 receptor-interactions

RECOMBINANT DNA TECHNOLOGY: Rearranging DNA molecules, manufacturing recombinant DNA. Recombinant DNA molecule constructed from segments obtained from different DNA molecules. P.34, 40, 83, 101, 116, 133, 155, 158, 159, 247 https://en.wikipedia.org/wiki/Recombinant_DNA

RECOMBINATION: Genetic recombination. Interchange of chromosomal parts or genes. Breaking and rejoining DNA strands, forming new DNA molecules. https://en.wikipedia.org/wiki/Genetic_recombination https://www.nature.com/scitable/topicpage/ dna-is-constantly-changing-through-the-process-6524876

RECTOCELE: Bulging of the anterior wall of the rectum into the posterior wall of the vagina. P.234

https://www.ncbi.nlm.nih.gov/pmc/articles/
PMC2967328/

REGENERATIVE MEDICINE: Creation of new organs,
tissues, and body parts from stem cells, which are placed
on a dissolvable matrix: tissue engineering, along with
self-healing by the body's systems. P.39
http://www.nature.com/articles/npjregenmed20167
https://www.nature.com/articles/s41536-017-0008-1?WT.
mc_id=EMI_RegMed_1704&spMailingID=53890539&
spUserID=MTc3MDI4ODk5NQS2&spJobID=114328
https://www.nature.com/articles/npjregenmed20167?
WT.mc_id=EMI_RegMed_1706&spMailingID=54243481&
spUserID=MTc3MDI4ODk5NQS2&spJobID=1181517

REJECTION: HOST VS GRAFT: Immunologic response
by organ recipient to allograft, damaging it. Immune
cells in the transplanted organ can also attack the host:
Graft vs. host response. P.41, 45, 71, 251, 270
http://emedicine.medscape.com/article/430449-over-
view#a4

RENIN: Proteolytic enzyme elaborated by juxtaglomerular cells of the kidneys that acts on angiotensin. P.75
https://www.britannica.com/science/
renin-angiotensin-system

RENIN-ANGIOTENSIN SYSTEM: RAS. A mechanism
of acute renal hypertension. Renal artery compression

or occlusion causing ischemia of the renal cortex results in renal juxtaglomerular cells converting prorenin into renin . Renin acts on angiotensinogen in the bloodstream from the liver, converting it to angiotensin I, which is converted to angiotensin II by angiotensin-converting enzyme. Angiotensin II acts on aldosterone producing cells in the adrenal cortex, causing aldosterone production, leading to sodium retention and increased plasma volume. This leads to an increase in blood pressure, and increased blood flow, including to the kidneys, resulting in stretching of renal afferent arterioles, giving negative feedback so that renin secretion tends to return towards normal. Renin-angiotensin systems are present in various other tissues, in addition to the kidneys.
http://www.ncbi.nlm.nih.gov/pubmed/17878513

REPROGRAMMING: (Cellular Reprogramming): Using the expression of four genes (**Yamanaka Factors**) to convert any cell into **induced pluripotent stem cells (iPSCs)**
https://www.salk.edu/news-release/turning-back-time-salk-scientists-reverse-signs-aging/
http://www.cell.com/cell/fulltext/S0092-8674(16)31664-6

RESVERATROL: Polyphenolic compound in red wine that may be partly responsible for the beneficial cardiovascular effects that have been attributed to red wine http://lpi.oregonstate.edu/mic/dietary-factors/phyto-chemicals/resveratrol

RETICULOENDOTHELIAL SYSTEM, also called: **MONONUCLEAR PHAGOCYTE SYSTEM (MPS):** Widespread system in reticular (thin banding fibers) connective tissue that forms antibodies to counteract foreign antigens. P.253
https://en.wikipedia.org/wiki/Mononuclear_phagocyte_system

RETINOPATHY: Disease of the retina . P.265
http://www.ncbi.nlm.nih.gov/pmc/articles/PMC3874488/

RH ISOIMMUNIZATION: Immune response of Rh Negative mother to her Rh positive fetus. First Rh positive child usually not affected. P.254
http://emedicine.medscape.com/article/797150-overview

RIBOSOME: The protein manufacturing machine. Complex molecular machine one millionth of an inch in diameter. Tiny organ (organelle)in the cytoplasm of the cell. Made up of proteins and ribosomal RNA (rRna)- the active component in protein synthesis. At the ribosome, the genetic code is read and translated into proteins. Amino acids are carried to the ribosome by transfer RNA (tRNA) . The genetic code instructions for making a protein are carried to the ribosome by messenger RNA (mRNA) from the DNA in the cell nucleus. At the ribosome, the tRNA recognizes the sequence of the genetic code on the mRNA and lines up the amino acids in the proper order. The ribosome catalyzes the formation of bonds between the amino acids. https://micro.magnet.fsu.edu/cells/ribosomes/ribosomes.html

RNA: Ribonucleic acid. Messenger RNA (mRNA) is essentially a copy of a piece of one strand of DNA. Proteins are not made from the DNA of the gene. A template of RNA is made from the gene DNA. The RNA is then processed. The processing involves splicing of RNA. This spliced RNA , the template upon which the protein is made (protein synthesis), is called messenger RNA (mRNA). mRNA goes to the ribosome in the cell cytoplasm, where it meets the transfer RNA (tRNA) carrying the amino acids. Under the influence of ribosomal RNA (rRNA), the amino acids are bound together to form the protein (see Ribosome). http://www.nature.com/scitable/definition/ribonucleic-acid-rna-45

ROBOTICS: A robot is a machine capable of automatically carrying out complex actions , programmable by computer. **Robotic surgery** is carried out via robotic telemanipulation. The surgeon's movements at a console are translated to surgical instruments previously placed into the patient

by minimally invasive technique. P.XII, 3, 82, 269
http://allaboutroboticsurgery.com/surgicalrobots.html

SARCOMA: A virulent form of malignant, solid tumor.
P, 117, 137, 145
http://sarcomahelp.org/reviews/who-classification-sar-comas.html

SARS: Severe acute respiratory syndrome. P.XV
http://www.cdc.gov/sars/about/fs-sars.html

SCAR: Cicatrix. Connective tissue in which fibroblasts
form granulation tissue. Older scars are composed of
dense collagenous tissue. P.384

SCURVY: Disease caused by lack of Vitamin C (ascorbic
acid). P.298
http://www.medicalnewstoday.com/articles/155758.php

SELF-DESTRUCT GENES: Genes that cause cell death
(apoptosis). P.VII, 18
http://www.nature.com/mt/journal/v23/n9/full/
mt2015139a.html

SENOLYTICS: Drugs that kill **senescent**, non-dividing
cells that accumulate in aging organs.
https://www.nature.com/news/to-stay-young-kill-zom-bie-cells-1.22872?WT.ec_id=NEWS-20171026&spMailin-gID=55224149&spUserID=MTc2NjY4OTM5NgS2&s
http://www.cell.com/cell/fulltext/S0092-8674(17)30246-5

https://www.ncbi.nlm.nih.gov/pubmed/22048312
https://www.ncbi.nlm.nih.gov/labs/journals/j-am-geri-atr-soc/new/2017-09-05/
http://onlinelibrary.wiley.com/wol1/doi/10.1111/jgs.14969
/full

SENSITIVITY: (In medical testing) Probability that a test result will be positive when the disease is present.
https://www.medcalc.org/calc/diagnostic_test.php

SEPSIS: Systemic inflammatory response to infection. P.357
http://www.ncbi.nlm.nih.gov/pmc/articles/PMC3684427/

Consensus Definitions for Sepsis and Septic Shock |
Critical Care Medicine | JAMA | The JAMA Network

SERM: Specific estrogen receptor modulator. A class of drugs used during the menopause to prevent osteoporosis. Some drugs in this class are protective against the formation of breast cancer. P.109, 113, 205, 327, 330
http://www.ncbi.nlm.nih.gov/pmc/articles/PMC3624793/

SEROTONIN: 5HT. 5-hydroxytryptamine. A monoamine neurotransmitter derived from tryptophan. P.195, 216
https://en.wikipedia.org/wiki/Serotonin

SEROTONIN/NOREPINEPHRINE REUPTAKE INHIBITORS: SNRI'S. Medications used in depression. P.216, 235. See: The Care of the Older Person: An Overview of Late-Life Depression: Artin Mahdanian,

Silvia Monti De Flores.
http://pharmacologycorner.com/serotonin-5ht-receptors-agonists-antagonist/#serotonin%20agonists

SHBG: Sex hormone binding globulin. Protein elaborated in the liver that binds and transports testosterone, dihydrotestosterone (DHT), and estradiol as inactive forms in blood. P.204
https://en.wikipedia.org/wiki/Sex_hormone-binding_globulin

SHINGLES: Delayed cutaneous manifestation by **Herpes Zoster** (Varicella: chicken pox) virus. Preventive vaccine available.
http://annals.org/aim/fullarticle/2671913/recommended-immunization-schedule-adults-aged-19-years-older-united-states
http://bmjopen.bmj.com/content/4/6/e004833

SIALOMUCIN: Mucopolysaccharide containing sialic acid. Component of lung airway secretion. P.254
http://www.ncbi.nlm.nih.gov/gene/8763

SIGNAL TRANSDUCTION (CELL SIGNALING): Transmission of molecular signals from cell surface receptors to the cell interior.
https://www.tocris.com/pharmacologicalBrowser.php?ItemId=187888#.V8hjh7ZTFwE

SINGLE CELL BIOLOGY: The study of the individual cell.
https://genomebiology.biomedcentral.com/articles
/10.1186/s13059-016-0941-0
http://www.nature.com/news/single-cell-biology-1.22241

SIRTUIN GENES: Genes that exert anti-aging effect in yeast. Increased sirtuin activity may be related to the mechanism by which caloric restriction extends life span.
https://www.ncbi.nlm.nih.gov/pubmed/18419308

SOMATIC CELL NUCLEAR TRANSFER: Therapeutic cloning. Nucleus is taken from an adult cell, and placed into an ovum whose own nucleus has been removed. These embryonic stem cells are induced to form specialized cells needed by the adult from whom the adult cell nucleus was taken.
http://www.hhmi.org/biointeractive/
somatic-cell-nuclear-transfer-animation

SPECIFICITY:(In medical testing) Probability that a test result will be negative when the disease is not present.
https://www.medcalc.org/calc/diagnostic_test.php

SPERMATOZOON: The male germ (sex) cell, derived from the testicle. It has a head, body and tail, and is motile. The spermatozoon swims up the female reproductive tract, eventually fertilizing (fusing with) the egg (ovum) in the fallopian tube.
https://www.boundless.com/physiology/textbooks/

boundless-anatomy-and-physiology-textbook/the-repro-
ductive-system-27/physiology-of-the-male-reproductive-
system-253/spermatogenesis-1234-9350/

SPINDLE NUCLEAR TRANSFER: Removal of the
nuclear spindle from a maternal oocyte and transferring
that spindle to a donor oocyte from which the spindle
has been removed, in order to obviate a mitochondrial
mutation . The donor oocyte containing the maternal
nuclear spindle is then fertilized.
https://www.ncbi.nlm.nih.gov/pmc/articles/PMC4005382/
https://www.sciencenews.org/blog/science-
ticker/first-%E2%80%98three-parent-baby%
E2%80%99-born-nuclear-transfer

SPLICING: The reattaching of the two ends of a stringlike material, after a piece has been removed. In **GENE
SPLICING,** DNA is cut and a gene inserted.
http://www.premierbiosoft.com/tech_notes/gene-splic-
ing.html

SSRI: Selective serotonin reuptake inhibitor. Medications
used in depression. P.194, 216. See: The Care of the Older
Person: An Overview of Late-Life Depression; Artin
Mahdanian, Silvia Monti De Flores
http://www.rxlist.com/the_comprehensive_list_of_anti-
depressants-page2/drugs-condition.htm#ssris

STATINS: Drugs that reduce circulating LDL (low density lipoprotein) by encouraging the LDL receptor to increase uptake. Decreased production of LDL-C (low density lipoprotein cholesterol) results. P.67, 79, 211
https://www.drugs.com/drug-class/hmg-coa-reductase-inhibitors.html

STEM CELL: An undifferentiated cell that has the potential to become a specialized cell with a specific function, such as a blood cell or a muscle cell. P.VIII, 39, 41, 43, 46, 47, 48, 64, 384
http://stemcells.nih.gov/info/basics/1.htm
http://fhs.mcmaster.ca/main/news/news_2016/life_saving_blood_stem_cells.html

STEM CELL TRANSPLANT: Injection of stem cells into the body to replace damaged or diseased tissue, blood. P.IX, 46
http://www.cancer.gov/about-cancer/treatment/types/stem-cell-transplant
http://journal.frontiersin.org/article/10.3389/fimmu.2016.00470/full

STENT: Self expanding tube placed in a blood vessel to keep that vessel patent. May be drug-eluting. P.81
https://www.sciencedaily.com/releases/2015/03/150316135610.htm

STEREOTACTIC RADIOSURGERY: SRS. Precisely focused radiation to scar and close the blood vessels of an arteriovenous malformation (AVM) in the brain. P.271 http://www.irsa.org/radiosurgery.html

STEREOTAXIS: Method in neurosurgery for locating points within the brain using an external three dimensional frame. P.112, 181

STROKE: Cerebrovascular accident. Damage to the brain by a blood clot in a vessel supplying the brain, or by hemorrhage into the brain. P.62, 73, 74, 84, 174, 178, 200, 203, 224, 266, 298, 327 http://www.neurology.org/content/early/2016/09/16/WNL.0000000000003238.abstract http://www.empr.com/news/repatha-heart-attack-stroke-prevention-pcsk9-inhibitor/article/711332 /?DCMP=EMC-MPR_DailyDose_cp_20171204& cpn=obgyn_all&hmSubId=&hmEmail=hIe6 FnTBLUDNqAesd8d7sd9Sz-y1cfMN0&NID=1538223656& c_id=&dl=0&spMailingID=18599771&spUserID= MTgxMDk3OTQyMDM0S0&spJobID=1160335565&spReportId=MTE2MDMzNTU2NQS2 http://www.acc.org/latest-in-cardiology/ten-points-to-remember/2018/01/29/12/45 /2018-guidelines-for-the-early-management-of-stroke

SUBUNIT: Ribosomal nucleic acid (rRNA) molecules (see "Ribosome")

http://www.microbe.net/simple-guides/fact-sheet-ribo-somal-rna-rrna-the-details/

SUDDEN INFANT DEATH SYNDROME: SIDS, Unexplained death during sleep of a seemingly healthy baby. P.260
http://emedicine.medscape.com/article/804412-overview

SUICIDE: Intentional, voluntary taking of own life. Contributory factor influencing average lifespan. P.9, 31, 97, 178, 194, 215, 216, 235
http://healthjournalism.org/blog/2014/04/exploring-risk-factors-rates-of-suicide-in-seniors/

SUPERAGER: Person 80 years or older with episodic memory ability at least as good as average middle-age adult. Significantly thicker brain cortex than same-age peers.
http://jamanetwork.com/journals/jama/article-abstract/2614177

T-LYMPHOCYTE: T-Cell. White blood cell that is immunologically competent. Responsible for cell-mediated immunity. Can attack surface antigens on malignant cells, if activated by prior presentation of the antigen. P.267
https://en.wikipedia.org/wiki/T_cell
https://www.frontiersin.org/articles/10.3389/fimmu.2018.00233/full?utm_source=F-AAE&utm_

medium=EMLF&utm_campaign=MRK_554072_35_
Immuno_20180227_arts_A

TALENS: Transcription Activator-Like Effector Nucleases.
Utilized to alter genes. See **Transcription, Nuclease.**
https://www.ncbi.nlm.nih.gov/pmc/articles/PMC3547402/

TARGETED AREA CORRECTION SEQUENCING:
Detection of mutations and rearrangements indicative of
cancer in cell-free plasma DNA.
https://www.ncbi.nlm.nih.gov/pmc/articles/
PMC4755822/
http://journals.plos.org/plosgenetics/article?id=10.1371/
journal.pgen.1005816
http://journals.plos.org/plosone/article?id=10.1371/jour-
nal.pone.0064271
http://journals.plos.org/plosgenetics/article?id=10.1371/
journal.pgen.1005816

TARGETED THERAPY: Drug designed to reverse the
effects of a specific mutation
http://www.ncbi.nlm.nih.gov/pubmed/23470539

TELOMERASE: Enzyme that maintains and repairs the
telomere.
http://study.com/academy/lesson/what-is-telomerase-
definition-function-structure.html

TELOMERE: The end of a chromosome. It is made up
of DNA. The telomere gives stability to the end of the

chromosome, preventing abnormal recombinations (mutations). The Care of the Older Person: Introduction: Jose Morais. P.VIII, 18, 34

https://en.wikipedia.org/wiki/Telomere
https://link.springer.com/article/10.1007/s10815-017-0967-6/fulltext.html?wt_mc=alerts.TOCjournals

TEMPLATE: The pattern from which copies are made.
https://engineering.ucsb.edu/~shell/che170/DNA-notes.pdf

TESTIS: The male gonad. P.247
http://emedicine.medscape.com/article/1949259-overview

TESTOSTERONE: The prominent androgen in the male. Male sex hormone. Present in lesser amounts in women. P.224, 244
http://www.livescience.com/38963-testosterone.html

THALLIUM STRESS TEST: Radioisotope uptake monitoring and myocardial perfusion assessment while patient is on a treadmill. P. 69, 331
http://pubs.rsna.org/doi/full/10.1148/rg.317115090

THROMBOPHLEBITIS: Inflammation of the wall of a vein in conjunction with thrombosis. P.203

THROMBOSIS: Blood clotting in a blood vessel. P.89, 109, 192, 199, 204, 255

THYMUS GLAND: Lymphoid gland of the immune system located in the neck that produces T-Cells. P.253, 267
http://biology.about.com/od/anatomy/ss/thymus.htm

TIA: Transient ischemic arteriospasm. Constriction of blood vessels in the brain with no permanent damage. P.86

TISSUE ENGINEERING: Combining cells, scaffolds, and biologically active molecules to create new tissue. P.384
https://www.nibib.nih.gov/science-education/science-topics/tissue-engineering-and-regenerative-medicine

TISSUE TYPING: Tissue antigens of prospective organ donor and recipient compared for histocompatibility. HLA (human leukocyte antigen) typing. P.45, 251, 270
http://www.encyclopedia.com/topic/Tissue_Typing.aspx

TOTIPOTENTIALITY: Capability of a cell to differentiate into unlimited number of cell types. P.43, 139
http://medical-dictionary.thefreedictionary.com/totipotential+cell

TOXEMIA: The hypertensive disorders of pregnancy. P.264

TPA: Tissue plasminogen activator. Protein involved in the breakdown of blood clots. P.83, 85
http://pharmacologycorner.com/thrombolytic-agents-mechanism-of-action-indications-contraindications-and-

side-effects/
http://atvb.ahajournals.org/content/29/8/1151.full

TRABECULA: Supporting structures of connective tissue. P.206

TRANSCRIPTION: Transfer of genetic code information between nucleic acids. The process by which the genetic code on the DNA gets into the mRNA template (see DNA, RNA).

http://www.vcbio.science.ru.nl/en/virtuallessons/cellcycle/trans/

TRANSCRIPTOME: Gene readouts (transcripts) of all the DNA in a cell by RNA
https://www.genome.gov/13014330/transcriptome-factsheet/

TRANSFORMATION ZONE: The outer cervix is lined by squamous cells, much like the vaginal lining. The inner canal of the cervix is lined by tall cylindrical cells. Where these two layers meet, there is an area of microscopic activity where the cylindrical columnar cells are being transformed, or over-ridden, by squamous cells. This is a benign process called **squamous metaplasia**. This area is called the transformation zone. It is in this area of cell activity that cancer of the cervix most commonly arises. P.132

TRANSLATION: The process by which the genetic code of mRNA becomes proteins.
https://bioweb.uwlax.edu/GenWeb/Molecular/Theory/Translation/translation.htm

TRANSLATIONAL MEDICINE: Mechanisms by which new drugs and tests get from the laboratory into the hands of physicians for administration to patients, and the mechanisms for ensuring that patients get necessary, services.
https://www.ncbi.nlm.nih.gov/pmc/articles/PMC2829707/
http://www.medscape.com/viewarticle/871305
nlid=110427_2581&src=WNL_mdplsnews_161104_msc-pedit_obgy&uac=66536PR&spon=16&impID=1228473&faf=1

TRANSPLANTATION: Transfer of organ or tissue from one individual to another. P.IX, 43, 44, 70, 251, 257, 270, 356
http://www.ajog.org/article/0002-9378(70)90382-0/abstract?cc=y=
http://www.who.int/transplantation/organ/en/

TRIGEMINAL NERVE: The fifth cranial nerve. P.195
http://emedicine.medscape.com/article/1873373-overview

TRIGLYCERIDE: Ester formed from glycerol and three molecules of fatty acids. P.154, 156, 157, 159
https://en.wikipedia.org/wiki/Triglyceride

TRIPTANS: Serotonin (5HT) receptor agonists. Medications that constrict blood vessels in the brain and are used in the treatment of migraine. P.198 http://archneur.jamanetwork.com/article.aspx?articleid=782346

TROPHOBLAST: Outer ring of cells around the blastocyst cavity that becomes the placenta. P.251, 254, 255 http://discovery.lifemapsc.com/in-vivo-development/trophoblast/trophoblast

TUBERCULOSIS: Infectious disease especially affecting the lungs caused by mycobacterium tuberculosis. P. 25, 262 http://www.thelancet.com/journals/lanres/article/PIIS2213-2600(15)00063-6/abstract

TUMOR: Abnormal growth . May be benign or malignant.

TUMOR GRADE: Appearance, abnormality of malignant tumor cells. P.100 https://www.cancer.gov/about-cancer/diagnosis-staging/prognosis/tumor-grade-fact-sheet

TUMOR SPECIFIC ANTIGEN (TSA): Protein or other molecule produced in tumor cells that sets off an immune response in the host. Used as tumor markers to identify tumor cells in the body. Used in the immunologic treatment of cancer. Also, **Tumor Associated Antigens (TAA)** that are significantly more abundant in cancer cells than in other tissue. TSA Definition CEA

Antigen, Prostate-Specific Antigen, CA125, CA19-9
https://www.researchgate.net/publication/9314460_
Demonstration_of_TumorSpecific_Antigens_in_Human_
Colonic_Carcinomata_by_Immunological_Tolerance_
and_Absorption_Techniques
https://www.researchgate.net/publication/12453745_
Self_recognition_in_the_Ig_superfamily_Identification_
of_precise_subdomains_in_carcinoembryonic_antigen_
required_for_intercellular_adhesion

TUMOR STAGE: Extent of the malignant tumor: its size
and spread.
https://www.cancer.gov/about-cancer/diagnosis-staging
/staging

TUMOR SUPPRESSOR GENE (Antioncogene): Genes,
such as the TP59 gene, that elaborate tumor suppressor proteins that control cell growth. Mutations (DNA
changes) in these genes are associated with cancer.
Tumor Protein 53 (TP53) that also has a role in germ cell
survival, is another example.
https://www.cancer.gov/publications/dictionaries/can-
cer-terms?cdrid=46657
https://www.nature.com/articles/d41586-017-07291-9?
WT.ec_id=NEWSDAILY-20171123&utm_source=
briefing&utm_medium=email&utm_campaig
http://www.fertstert.org/article/S0015-0282(17)32096-4
/fulltext?elsca1=etoc&elsca2=email&

elsca3=0015-0282_201801_109_1_&elsca4=
Obstetrics%20and%20Gyn

TURBINATES: Shelves of bone covered by thick mucous
membrane that project into the nasal passages. P.321
http://emedicine.medscape.com/article/874771-overview

UBIQUITIN-PROTEASOME SYSTEM : A protein
clearance mechanism with implications in aging and
age-related diseases
https://link.springer.com/article/10.1007/s10815-016-
0842-x?wt_mc=alerts.TOCjournals
http://www.nature.com/ncomms/2014/141208/
ncomms6659/fig_tab/ncomms6659_F1.html

ULTRASONOGRAPHY: Imaging by reflecting high
energy "sound" waves off objects. The waves have higher
frequency than sound that can be heard by humans. Four
dimensional sonography refers to images being seen in
real time. P.55, 112, 135, 136, 138, 141, 142, 194, 247, 330, 332
https://www.ncbi.nlm.nih.gov/pubmed/20541656
http://medical-dictionary.thefreedictionary.com/
ultrasonography

ULTRAVIOLET RAYS: UV. Short wavelength solar rays
that are invisible to the human eye. P.389
http://medical-dictionary.thefreedictionary.com/ultravi-
olet+rays

UMBILICAL CORD: The cord that connects the developing fetus to the placenta. Blood circulates in the cord via two arteries and one vein: the umbilical vein carrying nutrients and oxygen from the placenta to the fetus, and the umbilical arteries carrying waste products of metabolism and carbon dioxide away from the fetus, back to the placenta. P.252
https://www.ncbi.nlm.nih.gov/books/NBK53254/

UMBILICAL CORD BLOOD: Fetal blood that circulates via the umbilical cord. P. IX, 42
http://www.webmd.com/parenting/baby/features/
banking-your-babys-cord-blood#1
http://journal.frontiersin.org/article/10.3389/
fimmu.2017.00087/full?utm_source=newsletter&utm_
medium=email&utm_campaign=Immunology-w6-2017
https://www.nature.com/nature/journal/vaop/ncurrent
/full/nature22067.html

URETHRA: The passage from the urinary bladder to the vulva in the female, and to the penile meatus in the male. P.123

URETHROCELE: Bulging of the urethra into the anterior vaginal wall. P.234

URINARY INCONTINENCE: Involuntary loss of urine. Stress incontinence, urgency incontinence and neurogenic incontinence are types. P.234, 235, 237 See: The

Care of the Older Person: Incontinence In Older Adults:
Samer Shamout, Lysanne Campeau
http://jamanetwork.com/journals/jama/article-abstract
/2595508

UTERUS: The womb. Its endometrial lining undergoes
decidual change to receive the implanting fertilized egg
(zygote). During labor, muscular rhythmic contractions
of the uterine wall gradually send the fetus through the
birth canal. P.124, 265

VACCINE: Usually a killed, or attenuated (variant)
virus given by mouth or injection to activate the body's
immune system against the actual dangerous virus. If a
vaccinated person comes in contact with the actual virus,
the person's activated immune system kills the virus
before it can cause harm. Anticancer vaccines that target
malignant cells are now being developed and are in use.
P.20, 26, 37, 116, 121, 133, 148, 262, 267, 331
https://www.jci.org/articles/view/80009
http://journal.frontiersin.org/article/10.3389/
fimmu.2017.00800/full?utm_source=F-AAE&utm_
medium=EMLF&utm_campaign=MRK_333189_35_
Immuno_20170720_arts_A

VAGINA: The female genital canal leading from the
vulva to the uterus. Closed at rest, with the anterior
wall resting on the posterior wall. Its muscular, elastic
wall is lined by a mucous membrane that has a normal

secretion. The cervix protrudes through the vaginal vault. P.124

VALUE-BASED MEDICAL CARE: Quality of care relative to its cost. Quality is assessed in the areas of outcomes, safety and service. Outcomes includes measurement of mortality rates, complications, and resultant functional status of patients. Safety includes attention to infection rates, accidental falls, and medication errors. Service assesses patient satisfaction, wait times, access to treatment and procedures, and affordability. https://wire.ama-assn.org/education/value-based-care-elusive-concept-enters-curriculum?&utm_source=BHClistID&utm_medium=BulletinHealthCare&utm_term=120616&utm_content=MorningRounds&utm_campaign=BHCMessageID http://jamanetwork.com/journals/jama/fullarticle/2594716

VARICOSE VEINS: Veins that bulge out due to damage to their valves. P.89 http://emedicine.medscape.com/article/462579-treatment

VASOPRESSIN: Antidiuretic hormone (**ADH**). Formed in the hypothalamus and released from the posterior pituitary. Acts on renal collecting system, increasing water permeability and decreasing urine formation. Acts on vascular smooth muscle, causing vasoconstriction. http://www.cvphysiology.com/Blood%20Pressure/BP016

VEGETATIVE SYMPTOMS: Disturbances of functions necessary to maintain life: See: The Care of the Older Person: An Overview of Late-Life Depression: Artin Mahdanian, Silvia Monti De Flores. https://en.wikipedia.org/wiki/Vegetative_symptoms

VEGF: Vascular Endothelial Growth Factor. Angiogenic factor that promotes growth in vascular endothelial cells. Has a role in tumor angiogenesis. P.43, 384 http://www.nature.com/nrc/journal/v8/n8/full/nrc2403.html http://perspectivesinmedicine.cshlp.org/content/2/10/a006577.full

VEIN: A blood vessel that carries blood from the body towards the heart, usually transporting carbon dioxide and waste products of metabolism. Exceptions include the pulmonary vein, which carries oxygenated blood from the lungs to the heart for redistribution throughout the body, and the umbilical vein in the fetus, which carries oxygenated blood from the placenta to the fetal heart for redistribution throughout the fetal body .

VILLUS: A tiny projection from a surface P.252

VIRUS: An infecting agent so small that it cannot be seen under a light microscope. Viruses are made up of DNA or RNA. They can only replicate (divide) by invading into a host cell, and causing that cell to manufacture

more virus. P.XIII, 20, 130, 148
http://www.ncbi.nlm.nih.gov/books/NBK21523/

VITAL ORGAN: Organ necessary for life, including the heart, lungs, brain, kidneys and liver. P.44

VITAMIN: A substance that in small amounts is essential to metabolism, that naturally occurs in food. The Care of the Older Person: Could My Patient Be Malnourished ? : Jose Morais. P.275, 278, 295, 297
http://annals.org/article.aspx?articleid=1767855

VULVA: The female external genitalia. Includes: labia majora, labia minora, clitoris, vestibule, urethral orifice, mons pubis. P.123

WEST NILE VIRUS: A mosquito borne flavivirus that can cause encephalitis and meningitis. P.261, 319
http://www.cdc.gov/westnile/symptoms/

YAMANAKA FACTORS: Four genes that are important in cellular reprogramming to pluripotent stem cells.
https://www.ncbi.nlm.nih.gov/pubmed/19030024

ZIKA VIRUS: Mosquito borne. The fetuses of infected pregnant women have an increased incidence of micro-cephaly. There is an increased incidence of Guillain-Barre Syndrome with flaccid paralysis. Ref: Yale School of Medicine News, 08/26/2016
http://www.bloomberg.com/news/articles/2016-08-19/

zika-may-cause-brain-damage-in-adults-too

http://www.contagionlive.com/news/zika-research-reveals-virus-may-negatively-impact-adult-neural-stem-cells?utm_source=Informz&utm_medium=Contagion+Live&utm_campaign=Contagion_Live_Trending_News_9-5-16

http://jamanetwork.com/journals/jama/fullarticle/2593701

https://www.mdlinx.com/obstetrics-gynecology/top-medical-news/article/2017/01/02/3?utm_source=in-house&utm_medium=message&utm_campaign=in-the-news-jan17

ZONA PELLUCIDA: The glycoprotein outer envelope of the ovum. P.253

http://www.ncbi.nlm.nih.gov/pubmed/10497324

ZYGOTE: Fertilization (fusion of ovum and spermatozoon) results in a new cell: the zygote, which has forty six chromosomes including either an X or Y chromosome from the spermatozoon, and an X chromosome from the ovum. The zygote is therefore either XX (female) or XY (male). The zygote develops to a blastocyst stage with an inner cell mass that becomes the embryo, a fluid filled blastocyst cavity, and an outer ring of cells around the blastocyst cavity called the trophoblast, which becomes the placenta. P.44

http://www.biology-online.org/dictionary/Zygote